AF606214

COMMUNITY HEALTH NURSING

EVOLUTION AND PROCESS

SECOND EDITION

COMMUNITY HEALTH NURSING

EVOLUTION AND PROCESS

CATHERINE W. TINKHAM, R.N., B.S., M.P.H.

Professor
Community Health Nursing Department
Boston University School of Nursing
Boston, Massachusetts

ELEANOR F. VOORHIES, B.A., R.N., M.N., M.A.

Professor and Chairman
Department of Nursing
Fitchburg State College
Fitchburg, Massachusetts

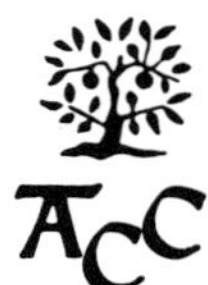

ACC

APPLETON-CENTURY-CROFTS / NEW YORK

Library of Congress Cataloging in Publication Data

Tinkham, Catherine W
Community health nursing.

Includes bibliographies and index.
1. Community health nursing—United States.
2. Nursing—Social aspects—United States. I. Voorhies, Eleanor F., joint author. II. Title.
RT98.T56 1977 610.73'43'0973 77-8120
ISBN 0-8385-1188-0

Copyright © 1977 by APPLETON-CENTURY-CROFTS
A Publishing Division of Prentice-Hall, Inc.

All rights reserved. This book, or any parts thereof, may not be used or reproduced in any manner without written permission. For information address Appleton-Century-Crofts, 292 Madison Avenue, New York, NY 10017.

77 78 79 80 81 / 10 9 8 7 6 5 4 3 2 1

Prentice-Hall International, Inc., London
Prentice-Hall of Australia, Pty. Ltd., Sydney
Prentice-Hall of India Private Limited, New Delhi
Prentice-Hall of Japan, Inc., Tokyo
Prentice-Hall of Southeast Asia (Pte.) Ltd., Singapore
Whitehall Books Ltd., Wellington, New Zealand

PRINTED IN THE UNITED STATES OF AMERICA

Cover design by Meryl Sussman Levavi

This book is dedicated to
OUR FORMER, PRESENT, AND FUTURE STUDENTS

PREFACE

Many events have occurred since the first edition was published. America has disentangled itself from an unpopular war in Vietnam and is still struggling with the postwar industrial and economic readjustment. The federal government, rocked by the Watergate scandal, has demonstrated its ability to endure and function effectively, in spite of a major crisis. The civil-rights movement has continued at a decelerated pace, while the women's-rights movement has gained momentum. The continuing developments in science and technology have resulted in undreamed-of progress, with breakthroughs in many areas of life today.

Nursing, an inherent part of this contemporary scene, has changed, developed, and grown in professional maturity. It has incorporated new knowledge and skills into its educational preparation and its practice, and has expanded its functions. It is more involved in political action and is consolidating its resources toward effecting change within the health-care system.

We are as firmly convinced as we were when we wrote the first edition that nursing must be increasingly knowledgeable about today's world and recognize and understand the effect of the ebb and flow of societal forces on its practices and responsibilities. It must further develop its own potential as one of the vital forces for a better life. We believe that nursing is firmly on this road. We also believe that our approach—community health nursing process—is realistic and enduring.

In revising we have made the following changes:

In Part I, Chapter 3 has been extended to cover the period from the New Deal through the mid-1970s. Major societal changes, as well as major changes in nursing, have been considered. Role expansion in nursing and the importance of competence in nursing practice is emphasized.

Chapter 4, "The Contemporary Scene," has been added. The focus is on issues that are of vital concern to nursing, with emphasis on community health nursing.

In Part II, an introduction has been added that sets the stage for Chapters 5 through 14. The content in each chapter has been expanded and/or revised, with further clarification of the relationship of knowledge to the community health nursing process. In each of the chapters there are substantial revisions. Chapter

14 has been completely rewritten. The bibliographies have been expanded and updated.

In Part III, we have again looked at the road ahead and have identified some of the challenges and pitfalls that nursing may encounter. We have also indicated the assets and vigor with which we believe community health nursing faces the future.

We are deeply grateful to our former and present students. Their critical thinking and thought-provoking questions have been a constant stimulus to us. The fact that students and community health nurses have found the book useful and valuable was a contributing factor in our decision to undertake the task of revision. We are also grateful to our colleagues and others who have used the book, for their comments, ideas, suggestions, and support. Last, but not least, each of us is grateful to the other–without whom neither the first nor the second edition would have been written.

C. W. T.
E. F. V.

PREFACE TO THE FIRST EDITION

We are living in exciting times in which the role and responsibilities of all the health professionals are being challenged. The people are demanding comprehensive health care while at the same time professional health workers are becoming more and more specialized, and their problems of communication are increasing. Everyone seems to have discovered the community as the base of operation. This has resulted in an increase in the services which are offered but a decrease in the coordination of these services. New kinds of health workers are appearing almost daily and others are being proposed. Health care is now considered a right to which all people are entitled regardless of their ability to pay.

Amidst all of this chaos, traditional public health and public health nursing programs are undergoing a metamorphosis. The artificial barriers between promotion of health and treatment of disease are disappearing. Emphasis is on the health of the community and how best to meet its health needs. A new partnership is developing in which health professionals from all disciplines and agencies must work together to provide the services demanded by the people. Community health nursing can no longer think of itself as having sole responsibility for nursing outside of the hospital but must work with other specialties within nursing and with other disciplines in order to better serve the people. The old relationships and strict agency prerogatives are no longer relevant. A new role for the community health nurse is evolving. It is imperative that she have the competencies and the vision to meet the challenge and make a contribution with others for improved and more comprehensive health services.

In order to better understand community health nursing today one must look to the past as well as to the present. Nursing, like other professions, did not chart its own course but was molded by the undulating forces of the times. It emerged and organized amidst turbulence and change; developed its own identity in a complex and dynamic society; and became a vital force in its own right. Early in the history of the profession, public health nursing became a specialty because of a need by the people for nursing care of the sick in their own homes. We believe that the overall developments in transportation, immigration and population, industrialization, science and technology, education, social consciousness, the role of government, and the role of women—separate though inexorably related—generated forces which were deciding factors in the evolution of nursing and public health nursing, and are still exerting their influences today. Each of these developments was not equally important simultaneously; however, their interrelatedness was and continues to be omnipresent. Some writers no doubt would select other events and resulting forces and interpret them differently, but we believe those which we have selected were instrumental in bringing about a whole new way of life which made it possible and inescapable for nursing and other professions to be nourished and to grow. Nursing must be increasingly knowledgeable about today's world and recognize and understand the effect of the ebb and flow of societal forces on its practices and responsibilities. It must further develop its own potential as one of the vital forces for a better life.

We have limited our exploration to developments in the United States. This book is divided into three parts—looking to the past, the present, and the future.

Part I includes three chapters. Chapter 1 deals with the period from 1865 to 1900. We have selected this period following the Civil War as our starting point because it was within this time that the seeds of organized nursing and public health nursing were about ready to burst forth. This was also the period within which the foundations were laid for many of our contemporary health programs and institutions.

Chapter 2 deals with the period from 1900 to the New Deal. It was during this time that organized nursing became viable and standards for education and practice were established. The responsibility of the government for the health of the people became apparent during these years.

Chapter 3 starts with the New Deal and goes through the Johnson era. This period was characterized by explosive developments in science and technology which drastically affected the way of life. Nursing became firmly established as a profession and great strides were made toward education of nurses within institutions of higher learning.

We have focused our attention on some of the changes which occurred in society during these three periods, and which we believe have influenced nursing and public health nursing. We have attempted to show implicitly or explicitly the interrelationships of these changes. What was America like at these times? How did public health nursing evolve as part of public health and as part of nursing? Why did it grow and organize as it did? What were some of the changes in education, in nursing education, and in the status of women which were significant to the development of nursing?

In Part II the major focus is on the process of community health nursing in relation to the family and the community. Forces in society will constantly change and affect the directions in which nursing with other professions will move. It is for this reason that we are emphasizing the process of nursing as we believe the process will remain essentially the same within a changing society.

The term "public health nursing" has been broadened to "community health nursing." This concept refocuses the nurses' concern for the health of the people and puts it where it belongs—in the community itself, thus removing the responsibility from the aegis of specific agencies. It involves the nurse with professional and nonprofessional persons in the community in a broadened and different kind of partnership. What is the relationship of public health nursing organizational patterns to the growing demands of the public for improved health care? What is the influence on community health nursing of the rapidly increasing governmental support of a variety of community health programs? What is the impact on community health nursing of the increased numbers of health workers who have recently discovered the community? What effect has the knowledge explosion had upon community health nursing? What is the relationship between traditional public health nursing services and the needs of a changing, mobile population?

In Part III, we have looked at the road ahead. We have identified some of the assets and liabilities with which community health nursing faces the future; have discussed its developing role as the family health nurse practitioner, and pointed out some of the challenges and pitfalls which undoubtedly lie ahead. Finally, we have indicated some of the implications for nursing education and research.

This book is planned for the use of nursing students in colleges and universities, and for community health nurse practitioners, as well as other community health workers.

We wish to express our thanks and appreciation to Marie Farrell, Dean Emeritus of the Boston University School of Nursing, for her perceptiveness, constructive criticism, and support; to our students who unknowingly have contributed many ideas; to Gertrude Smith, whose careful and meticulous work contributed immeasurably to the preparation of this manuscript; and finally, to each other, without whom this book would never have been written.

C.W.T.
E.F.V.

Contents

CHAPTER 1

THE PERIOD FROM 1865 TO 1900

THE SCENE AT THE CLOSE OF THE CIVIL WAR

We will start our exploration of the past by attempting to recapture some of the feelings and aspirations of the American people at the close of the Civil War. We recognize the limitations of this approach, as each person looking back over history will interpret events differently, depending upon his background and frame of reference. We will explore the environment in which the people lived: their growing cities; the teeming slums; the deplorable health conditions; the expanding transportation; and the burgeoning industry. We will identify some of the forces and changes which were shaping their way of life; the aftermath of the antislavery agitation; the changing role of women; and the strivings for education.

Although America after the war was primarily rural, cities were developing rapidly and bringing with them problems of housing, sanitation, and health. The population, 31,443,321 in 1860,[1] was growing because of immigration from northern and western Europe. Many of these newcomers settled in the crowded slums of the growing cities. This was still a horse-and-buggy era, and goods, passengers, mail, and all manner of things were transported across the country by stagecoach and Pony Express. Railroads were expanding, but they did not link the East with the West. The frontiers of the West were still being settled. The slavocracy of the agrarian South was dissolved and no longer a threat to the entire economy. Industry which, especially in the North, had geared itself to the war effort, was now ready to expand.

For a democracy to work there is a need for educated people; this was becoming more and more apparent, although only a few states had compulsory school attendance laws. The public school system was in its formative stages, and only a minority of the young people attended high school. In the large eastern cities boys and girls were educated separately. Outside the cities and in the West, where the population was sparse, they were educated together. By the close of the war, women had become accepted as the teachers of both boys and girls. Nowhere else in the world had this happened, and it was to have a profound effect on the development of college education for women. Higher education was predominately for men in private colleges which offered classical curricula with strong emphasis on theology. In 1862 Congress had passed the Morrill Act to make possible the establishment in each state of at least one college particularly adapted to the needs of agriculture and industry. The implications of this legislation had not yet become evident.

Women's place was in the home for the rearing and nurturing of children. The superiority of the male was stressed over and over again. Wives and children, along with other chattels, were the property of the husband. In most states married women could neither own property separately from their husbands nor decide about the disposition of property at their death. Women were not allowed to vote. Very few occupations were open to them. Pay for those who were employed was lower than that of men. Prior to the Civil War a few women, both individually and in groups, had actively participated in the rebellion against the system of slavery. They had become involved in public debates and lectures, and some had expressed their opinions in writing. Harriet Beecher Stowe's *Uncle Tom's Cabin* was widely read and had far-reaching effects. Some of the women in the South had freed their slaves and gone north to campaign against slavery. Paralleling this whole involvement of women in abolition was the beginning of the feminist movement, which was to gain momentum after the war and finally result in women's suffrage.

The winds of change affecting the status of women, which had arisen prior to the Civil War, were intensified by the war itself. Women had become involved in all aspects of the war effort and had taken over many of the jobs previously held by men. Their accomplishments had equaled and often exceeded those of men. It was largely through the efforts of the women in the North that the secretary of war, in 1861, approved a document that gave the president the power to appoint a United States Sanitary Commission to oversee the health and welfare of the army and to be a channel of communication between the people and the government.[2] The United States Sanitary Commission became the forerunner of the American Red Cross. Ladies' Aid societies were established in the northern states and were affiliated with the Commission. The women in the Aid Societies had involved themselves with the care of the sick and wounded soldiers, with the provision of supplies for the soldiers on the fighting front, and with the maintenance of contact between the soldiers and the home front. The contribution of these women is graphically described by Greenbie:

> One thing that universally impressed the many gentlemen whose time or money the Ladies' Aid societies commandeered was the "perfect attitude of women for business." By the end of the Civil War, this Sanitary Commission enterprise which the ladies had started, and of which they remained to the end the backbone, was worth about $50,000,000. And in those days that was a very large business enterprise, indeed. They had the cooperation of all railroads and express companies in transporting their stores free, and of the telegraph companies in sending their messages free. They had many and intricate arrangements for cooperation with the army. They had, in all, about 32,000 groups of women, large and small, organized as cooperating Ladies' Aids societies.
>
> To keep this vast network of business in any kind of order was a test of efficiency in detail and in overall organization to which the housewives of the land had risen nobly. As Dr. Bellows said in a message quoted, with endorsement by Limus P. Brockett, a merchant of New York, "A generous emulation among the branches of the United States Sanitary Commission, managed generally by women, usually, however, with some aid from men, brought their business habits and methods to an almost perfect finish. . . . They acknowledged and answered, endorsed and filed their letters; they sorted their stores and kept an accurate account of stock; they had their books and reports kept in the most approved forms; they balanced their cash accounts with the most painstaking precision; they exacted of each other regularity of attendance and punctiliousness of official etiquette." They did even more than this. They created and introduced into the government records the first complete clerical system any army had ever had. It was their careful registering of the soldiers that formed the basis of the pension system for Civil War veterans.[3]

The women who had been so totally involved in the war effort had found this a rewarding and satisfying experience. They had become less provincial and more nationalistic in their outlook and were loath to return to their former subordinate existence.

Many women and an increasing number of men were beginning to demand opportunities in higher education for women. Matthew Vassar had been tremendously impressed by the ability of women during the war. in 1865 he established Vassar College, which was the first college to provide education for women similar to that offered to men in men's colleges.

Health conditions were poor throughout the country, particularly in the crowded slums of the growing cities. The people were continuously plagued by illnesses of all kinds which they accepted as the way of life. Life expectancy at birth was about 41 years.[4] Tuberculosis was endemic and the leading cause of death. Epidemics of cholera, yellow fever, and scarlet fever were still sweeping the country, but were on the wane. The causes of disease were unknown and thought to be due to the environment. Thus, there was great emphasis on sanitation. Medical research was practically nonexistent even in the best medical centers. A few boards of health had been established in some of the cities, but there were no organized public health programs as we know them today.

Hospitals were considered pest houses and looked upon as places in which to die. Their patients were usually the poor and homeless. Nursing care was given by untrained, unqualified men and women who were predominantly from the poorer classes. They had servant or domestic status and were often recruited from the ranks of prisoners, scrubwomen, and convalescent patients. The majority of the sick were given care at home by female family members or neighbors, many of whom had a great deal of experience in caring for the sick and were respected members of their communities. Organized nursing had not as yet been established, but the influence of Florence Nightingale on the development of trained nurses in England was beginning to be felt in the United States.

There were stirrings of a social consciousness which was expressing itself in various ways and was to become full blown by the end of the century. Many of the women who had had experience as volunteer nurses in the army were anxious to use their knowledge in caring for the people at home. Literature, both fiction and nonfiction, was describing some of the contemporary social problems and making the people more aware of and concerned about the plight of the poor, the conditions of the slums, and the general poor health and sanitary conditions. Compassion for humanity, so sharply expressed through the abolitionist movement, was growing.

The federal government was fairly weak at this time and maintained a "hands off" policy except for some of the overall responsibilities that were specifically stated in the Constitution. Each state assumed major responsibility for its own affairs with little or no relationship to those of other states.

1865 TO 1900

The period from the close of the Civil War to the turn of the century was particularly significant in the history of the United States. It was a time of change and turmoil—no less dynamic than that with which we struggle today. It saw what had been a restless, bitterly divided country pick itself up, bind up its wounds, and go forward with hope and optimism for the future.

The Civil War, with all its horror and devastation, instead of dividing the country, proved to be a unifying force. Although the wounds were deep and bitter (and some would influence the people for generations) there was a national cohesiveness and sense of unity that had not been apparent before. The rapid expansions on all fronts that occurred between 1865 and 1900 had their beginnings before the war, but it was almost as if the war had unleashed the energies of the people and made it possible for them to move forward as a nation.

TRANSPORTATION

Some historians say that progress in transportation was the most important development during this period. In 1869 the completion of the transcontinental railroad linked the East and West for the first time. The results were profound and far-reaching. Great growth and settlement of the West was made possible, and by the end of the century the era of the frontiers was over. A more common culture began to develop. A letter mailed in New York, which formerly had taken weeks and even months by stage coach, or by the perilous voyage around the Isthmus of Panama, now reached the West Coast in a matter of days. Magazines, newspapers, and books were more readily available. Women in the West learned about fashions in the East, and the demand for dress patterns and materials grew. Housewives wanted to purchase new foods and household goods which were appearing in increasing numbers. A vast new market clamored for more and diverse machinery and equipment.

Towns sprang up almost overnight along the railroad routes and became centers for storage and transfer of produce from the large and small farms and factories throughout the land. Men sweated in great mills in Pittsburgh and other growing cities, and strained to produce coal and steel for the growing miles of railroad tracks and passenger and freight cars. Americans who previously had been isolated on small and large farms, particularly in the Middle and Far West, began to travel. Many sought work in and around the cities, which were teeming with businesses and opportunities. By 1900 there were 193,000 miles of railroad.[5] The building of the railroads was primarily a private enterprise. The situation was ripe for businessmen alert to rich opportunity. They were not found wanting. As the transcontinental lines developed, vast fortunes were made, large companies were formed, and later great mergers took place. The federal and state governments gave generous grants of land and financial loans to the railroad companies. This assistance, however, was often exploited by the states, many of whom passed legislation geared to their own interests, unrelated to and at times detrimental to those of other states. Because of these practices, which were of national concern, Congress passed the Interstate Commerce Act in 1887, which outlawed many of the discriminatory acts of the railroads. This was the first regulatory legislation passed by the federal government in the interests of society as a whole. Some say it heralded the beginning of the end of individualism in the United States.

The horse and buggy and, in the latter part of the century, the bicycle were the most common modes of transportation, in spite of the growth of the railroads. By 1900 the discovery of electricity had led to the development of trolley cars in the larger cities, and the first subway had been introduced in Boston. A few horseless carriages were appearing in the cities, but there was not much confidence in their future. Dulles quotes a writer of the times:

> "The ordinary 'horseless carriage'," it was pontifically stated by one editorial writer of the day, "is at present a luxury for the wealthy, and although its price will probably fall in the future, it will never, of course, come into common use."[6]

INDUSTRIALIZATION

Even though some say that developments in transportation were the most important at this time, the remarkable growth in transportation could not have occurred without the industrial know-how which accompanied it. Scientific and technologic advances made possible new products, equipment, and methods of production. The practical ingenuity of people in America, that is, the ability to apply the fruits of scientific discoveries, from both Europe and the United States, was one of their greatest assets. The discovery of electricity, the incandescent lamp, the telephone, the typewriter, and many other conveniences effected vast changes throughout the nation. Markets grew, not only in America, but in other countries as well. Industrial expansion was favored by rich, untapped natural resources, a ready labor force, investment of capital from abroad, absence of trade barriers, lack of hampering traditions, and the "hands off" policy of the federal government.

The industrial revolution, though primarily a phenomenon of cities, affected every corner of the country. It made possible the mechanization of farming and changed it from an individual occupation to a business venture. Between 1850 and 1900 the number of farm workers doubled, while the value of produce increased twentyfold.[7]

IMMIGRATION AND POPULATION

Industrialization could not have occurred without a ready supply of labor to meet the demands of industry and farming. In addition to the sons and daughters of farmers and businessmen, an endless flow of immigrants supplied the bulk of the migratory labor force of agriculture, lumber camps, and construction. Thousands upon thousands of workers poured into the cities to meet the demands of industry. According to Dulles,

> At the century's end, New York reported half as many Italians as Naples, as many Germans as Hamburg, as many Jews as Warsaw, and twice as many Irish as Dublin. The foreign-born in Chicago exceeded its total population of a decade earlier. Its busy streets were crowded with Germans, Swedes, Norwegians, Italians, Poles, Lithuanians, Hungarians, and Slovenes. And, in varying degrees, much the same could be said of other urban centers from Boston to St. Louis.[8]

Whole families were crowded into dark, damp, poorly ventilated rooms—often with no outside windows—which opened only onto sunless shafts. Plumbing facilities were antiquated or nonexistent and, of necessity, shared by many. Poorly constructed, overcrowded tenements, difficult to reach, made the danger of devastating fires imminent, and the ominous clanging firetruck was a frequent visitor. The sanitary and health conditions were intolerable. Tuberculosis, diphtheria, and venereal diseases were just a few of the many communicable diseases which were rampant. Poverty, overcrowding, and lack of recreational facilities furnished an environment in which crime and delinquency flourished. Public health measures were eminently inadequate to cope with such overwhelming problems. A growing concern about the environment in which people were living and the responsibility of the community for the protection of the individual was beginning to be apparent everywhere. Numerous books and articles graphically describing the intolerable living and working conditions of the people in the slums made their appearance. Publishing houses multiplied. The ranks of those concerned increased, fed by a growing middle class and a better educated and informed public. Reform groups organized and flourished. Many of these directed their energies toward the social-service and health fields.

As bad as the slum environment were the working conditions. Men, women, and children, separately and as family units, labored in dark, crowded, poorly ventilated shops and factories 10 to 12 hours a day, for six days a week—all for less than a living wage. It is difficult for us to understand why the situation was tolerated as long as it was. It was probably due to the fact that America was thought to be a land of promise and opportunity. A feeling of optimism prevailed. Anything was within the realm of possibility, if not for the parents, perhaps for the children. The very struggle for life itself was worth the rewards which might be ahead. Many immigrants were able to save money, buy small businesses, and improve their living and working conditions. The desire of these individuals to retain their freedom, to grasp any opportunity which might present itself, may account for the fact that sporadic attempts toward organization of workers into labor unions failed, for the most part, during this period.

The population expanded by leaps and bounds, doubled between 1870 and 1890, and by 1900 was 76,303,387.[9] By this time immigration had contributed 20 million newcomers.[10] In spite of the problems of the poor, America was predominantly a middle-class society, and this was expanding. Class structure was not rigid, and aspirations for upward mobility were high and often realized. The standard of living was improving, and families with higher incomes and better transportation were beginning to move out of the crowded cities and settle in the suburbs. In sharp contrast to the grinding poverty of some was the tremendous wealth of a small but increasing segment of the population. Men such as Andrew Carnegie, who exemplified the rags-to-riches heroes, felt they owed something to America for their good fortune. They gave huge sums to charity based on the philosophy of helping those who wished to help themselves. Thus, public philanthropy was begun by those men who had been able to make a great deal of money by utilizing the fruits of society and who wished to give back to society a portion of their money and some of the opportunities they had enjoyed.

EDUCATION

The concept of the value of education for all in a free society had been built into the very fabric of American life and was taking hold. Education gave hope and possibility for individual advancement, for solutions of society's complex problems, and for acquisition of new knowledge applicable to business and industry. The task of providing education for such a polyglot people seemed almost insurmountable. Most of the wealthy were educated privately; many of the poor, not at all. Middle-class children attended good and bad, large and small, public and private schools. Agitation for free public education persisted and grew. The federal government was supportive but left to the states the job of overseeing and regulating this heterogeneous system of education. By 1900 the average American had 1046 days of school, or more than twelve times as many as his great-grandfather.[11] Between 1870 and 1900 the number of high schools rose from 500 to 6,000.[12] However, less than 10 percent of the population reached high school, and less than 1 percent went to college.[13]

Reform was not limited to grammar and secondary school education. Well-established men's private colleges in the East were trying to create some sort of order out of the new conditions. They were tackling the problem of shaping an educational plan that would be as meaningful for their students as classical education had been for earlier students. They began to study and to revise their curricula, to de-emphasize preparation for the clergy, and to expand offerings in the humanities and in the sciences. State universities appeared in the West and made higher education available for both men and women. The western tradition of educating boys and girls together in grammar and high school carried over to university education.

There was a great difference of opinion, and controversy, over higher education for women. Some critics believed that sustained brain activity would drain away strength from child-bearing ability; college women desiring children would be incapable of safe and sound motherhood; and college education would ruin a girl's body instincts and unsex her. The severest critics, nevertheless, agreed that they would rather have educated than uneducated women teach their children. In spite of controversy, educational opportunities for women increased. Nothing could really have stopped it. The time was ripe and there were always people ready and eager to take up the challenge. Private women's colleges developed in the East where there was the tradition of private men's colleges. By June 1899, 14,824 women had earned a bachelor's degree. This was the largest number of educated women in any country in the world.[14]

In 1876 the first graduate school was established at Johns Hopkins University. By 1900 graduate education was becoming increasingly important, and was established, for the most part, within the graduate schools of the larger universities. Graduate professional education in law, medicine, theology, dentistry, and veterinary medicine increased. The percentage of women admitted to these schools showed a greater increase than that of men.

Many factors contributed to the development of higher education for both men and women. Not the least of these were the philosophy of individualism and the noninterfering role of the government. Men who had become wealthy as a result of the industrial revolution found a fruitful and satisfying outlet for their philanthropy in colleges and universities. By contributing to higher education they were also influencing the improvement of educational opportunities for their sons. The resources of a growing body of alumni also added to educational and financial support. High value was placed on scientific knowledge and its importance to technology, without which industrialization could not have occurred.

WOMEN

Perhaps one of the greatest changes occurred during this period in the status and role of women. The results of the industrial revolution, such as the development of the typewriter and need for clerical help, opened up new possibilities for women to work outside the home and to secure some measure of economic independence. The unquenchable thirst of the people for more goods created a constant need for workers to produce them, and many women wishing to supplement their family's income (inadequate because of low wages) moved into these jobs. By and large these women worked long hours and had little time or energy left over to become involved in the increasing concern over women's rights.

As a result of technical advances and an abundant supply of domestic help, a growing number of women in the upper and middle income levels were relieved of much of their household drudgery. Because of their social position, work outside the home was frowned upon, even though they were living in the midst of a bustling society in which work was considered a virtue. Some of these women exemplified the genteel, frail woman whose main mission in life was to amuse her husband. These were usually the ones who became the leaders and participants in the social activities of the times. Others were not satisfied with this role and became involved in a variety of education, health, social, and political reforms.

As the number of women with higher education grew, their influence was felt in many areas. Improved education for teachers was raising the level of instruction in public schools. Women authors were becoming abundant. Women participated in public debates and gave lectures on a variety of subjects. Women's organizations sprang up, and in 1889 the Federation of Women's Clubs was established. As the level of education improved and as the members became more aware of the society in which they lived, the programs of these organizations expanded and many became powerful forces in social and political reform.

The mobility of the population brought about a marked change in family life. Relatives who had previously lived in proximity to one another found themselves separated and living in unfamiliar surroundings. The authoritarian position of the husband and father was weakened as the wife assumed more responsibility for the caring and rearing of children, as well as for the economic support of the family. The birthrate was decreasing and divorce was on the rise.

The growing militancy of women for their right to vote gained momentous proportions. By 1900 women were voting in many local elections, and four western states had given equal suffrage to women.[15]

The increasing independence and growing participation of women in all facets of society were frowned upon by the majority of men and a large number of women. Many of the ills of society, such as the breakup of families, illegitimacy, the juvenile crime rate, and the increase in venereal disease were blamed on the fact that women were not at home where they belonged.

NURSING

Some of the women who had been involved in the Civil War had become friends with Florence Nightingale and had gone to England to observe the developments in the training school for nurses which she had established. Others began corresponding with her and were learning more about her philosophy of nursing. Her book, *Notes on Nursing,* had become more readily available to readers in the United States with the improved transportation, and many were using some of her methods in nursing their own family members. Some of the Ladies' Aid Societies that were established during the war had continued as organized groups and were involved in various philanthropic and charitable works. One of these, the State Charities Aid Association of New York, sponsored a study in 1872 of the care of patients at Bellevue Hospital. The deplorable state of the patients and the poor care they were receiving appalled and shocked the members. The Association was instrumental in bringing these intolerable conditions to the attention of the public. At the same time some of the technologic advances, such as the development of the sphygmomanometer and the hypodermic, were changing medical and nursing practice. The introduction of asepsis, new surgical techniques, and improved preoperative and postoperative care were demanding better prepared personnel and a new relationship between doctors and nurses. Physicians were becoming more and more concerned about the care their patients were receiving, and some gave individual and group instruction to the women who were nursing tlem. Women physicians were increasing in number and, because of the opposition against them, were particularly anxious to prove their worth. Some were personally involved in improving nursing care for their patients. In 1867 Dr. Marie Zakrzewska, who was professor of obstetrics at the New England Female Medical College in Boston, initiated a nursing program at the New England Hospital for Women and Children. This program later developed under the direction of Dr. Susan Dimock. Linda Richards successfully completed the program and received a diploma in 1872. She is often referred to as the first trained nurse in the United States.

A year later the first three modern training schools for nurses were established—one at Bellevue Hospital, one at New Haven Hospital, and the other at Massachusetts General Hospital. Each of these schools, using the model developed by Florence Nightingale, was established by lay groups who were financially independent of the hospital. However, due to lack of funds and strong opposition from the medical profession, they succumbed early to financial control by the hospital. Thus, the pattern of hospital control of nursing was established, and from then on training schools emerged at the whim of the individual hospitals.

There was considerable opposition from many sources to the new system of training schools for nurses, and fear was expressed that the nurses would be taught too much and think they knew more than the physicians. There was also apprehension that better-educated women would not enter the nursing schools and, if they did, would become disillusioned and leave nursing after they had been trained. However, it soon became evident that patients received better care when pupil nurses were available, that the death rate of patients in hospitals where there were pupils decreased, and that pupils were a cheap source of labor. As a result new hospitals developed, and the number of training schools for nurses increased by leaps and bounds.

The early schools of nursing grew up in a haphazard individualistic way with each hospital a law unto itself. There were no uniform admission standards, and pupils with eighth-grade education were taught together with college graduates. The length of the courses varied from 1 to 2 years. Pupils worked from 10 to 12 or more hours each day. There was no standard curriculum pattern, and classes were held irregularly in addition to the long work day. Militarylike discipline prevailed, with absolute obedience to the physician. Pupils lived in nurses' homes set up by the hospital and were socially isolated from the outside world. The overwhelming majority of the graduates went into private nursing, usually on a 24-hour-a-day basis. The hospitals were staffed entirely by pupil nurses, and the employment of staff nurses in the hospital was not even considered. The schools were organized to carry on the work of the hospitals and not to educate nurses.

In spite of these conditions women from the middle and upper income groups enrolled in the nursing schools, and there was no problem of recruitment. Apparently, the opportunity to care for the sick provided these women with a satisfying outlet for the idealism and humanitarianism so characteristic of nursing and the times. Nursing also opened up a whole new occupation for women whose opportunities had previously been limited primarily to teaching.

At the same time that nursing was getting deeper and deeper into the apprenticeship type of education, medical education was going in the opposite direction and beginning to give up the apprenticeship system. There was a movement toward medical schools becoming fully independent of the hospitals in which their students had experience, and setting up university hospitals under their own control.

By 1893 there were 225 schools of nursing,[16] and the number was growing. This rapid proliferation made it imperative that some common education standards be developed if nursing were to become a profession. Nursing, too, had women of imagination and vision who were ready and willing to take up the challenge. One of the outstanding ones was Isabel Hampton (Robb). She exemplified the eminent women who were the leaders in many of the contemporary social, educational, health, and political endeavors. She had a background of private school education, had received an upbringing characteristic of middle- and upper-class society, and had taught school before entering nursing. It was largely through her leadership that in 1893 the Society of Superintendents of Training Schools of Nurses of the United States and Canada was organized. According to Roberts,

> The primary purposes of the new society were to advance the best interest of the nursing profession by establishing and maintaining a universal standard of training, and by promoting fellowship among its members by meetings, papers, and discussions on nursing subjects and by interchange of opinions.[17]

This organization was later to become the National League for Nursing Education. The membership consisted primarily of administrators and directors of schools of nursing.

Two years later, the Nurses' Associated Alumnae Association of the United States and Canada, which later became the American Nurses' Association, was organized. It opened its membership to all alumnae of training schools for nurses and stated the following:

> The objects of this Association shall be to strengthen the union of nursing organizations; to elevate nursing education; to promote ethical standards in all the relations of the nursing profession.[18]

With the establishment of these two organizations, nursing had taken a giant step toward becoming a profession. There was now a medium by which nurses could develop criteria and standards for nursing practice and nursing education, could develop a code of ethics, and could meet together to discuss common problems and share new techniques and developments.

PUBLIC HEALTH NURSING

It was not until 1886, after the value of organized nursing care in the hospitals and the benefit of private nursing to patients in their own homes had been demonstrated, that organized district nursing developed. It was because of the success of private nursing of patients in upper- and middle-income levels that questions were raised about how to bring a similar type of service to the poor. At the same time application of the germ theory was laying groundwork for control of communicable disease. Poverty was beginning to be considered a result of social maladjustment; and there was a belief that the benefits of medicine and nursing should be available equally to the poor and the rich.

There had been sporadic attempts for many years to provide some nursing care to the sick poor in their homes. In many instances women had been employed by churches, guilds, settlement houses, dispensaries, and other charitable organizations to go into the home of the sick persons who were connected with the particular organization. However, these attempts, though laudable in their purposes, were not too successful. The women who were employed were not necessarily trained and did not always know how to give nursing care in the home, particularly when they were confronted with the many other problems of the people who lived in the slums. Nursing was often secondary to other purposes for visiting, and it was not clear what nursing care in the homes really included. Also, this early nursing service was mixed with charity and almsgiving, with bringing a religious message to the family, with being only a follow-up of the doctor's orders to the patient, and with being associated with a free dispensary. Nursing was not a primary focus for visiting, and the availability of nursing services to all the people in the community was not a goal of these early attempts.

The first organized district nursing began in 1886, and at first, according to Jacques,[19] the nurses merely followed the physicians' orders, gave some treatments, and recorded the temperature and pulse. However, this was much more than the patient had previously received, and the physician, patient, and family all looked upon this amount of professional care as a great advancement. The nurses very soon realized that because they were in the home for only a short time, in contrast to the private duty nurse, someone had to be taught to take care of the patient between the nurses' visits. Instruction to families about how to care for the patient naturally included personal hygiene, sanitary measures of the sick room, and aspects of healthful living for the entire family. Thus, almost from the very beginning, teaching and prevention became important functions of the district nurse.

The first district nursing associations, one in Boston and one in Philadelphia, were formed in the same year. Each developed in a different way and without any relationship to the other. However, both were organized by women who were inspired by the work of William Rathbone in England and who had investigated the organization of district nursing in Liverpool. In Boston two socially conscious women approached the Women's Education Association to support the work of a district nurse. They had to convince the Association that district nursing related mainly to education, in order for its sponsorship to be consistent with the other educational efforts of the Association. Thus, the title Instructive District Nursing was coined. The group then met with persons in the Boston Dispensary, which was providing free medical care to the sick poor and had divided the city into dispensary districts, to discuss how the two groups could work together. As a result, in February of 1886, one nurse was employed to work in one dispensary district. It was not long before other nurses were employed for the other districts. The nurse in each district was assigned to a physician and was responsible for carrying out medical orders. Sometimes the doctor and nurse would visit a patient together. The patients were not charged any fee for the service. Supervision was given by two lay managers of the association who were assigned to each district. It was not until 1900 that a nurse was employed to oversee the work and to supervise the nurses.

It was not long before the value of the work was well recognized, and in 1888 the Instructive District Nursing Association was incorporated and became an independent voluntary agency. The objects were:

> 1. To provide and support thoroughly trained nurses, who, acting under the immediate direction of the out-patient physician of the Boston Dispensary, shall care for the sick poor in their own homes instead of in hospitals.
> 2. By precept and example to give such instruction to the families which they are called upon to visit as shall enable them henceforth to take better care of themselves and their neighbors by observing the rules of wholesome living and by practicing the simple arts of domestic nursing.[20]

Probably the emphasis on teaching of the Boston organization was due in part to its early sponsorship by the Women's Education Association. However, the teaching function of the nurse had been stressed by Florence Nightingale and was one of the strengths of the early organizations.

At the same time that the work was being developed in Boston, a group of prominent women in Philadelphia, who had also been inspired by William Rathbone's work, organized and employed a nurse to give nursing to the sick at home. They were not sponsored or affiliated with any other group and at first had trouble finding patients. They only had $100 with which to start their venture and decided very early to charge the patients for the cost of the carfare of the nurse. It soon became evident, as the service became better known, that patients other than just the sick poor needed and wanted nursing service from the district nurse. As a result, they decided to charge the patient for the cost of the nursing visit. The Visiting Nurse Society of Philadelphia was incorporated in 1887. The purpose was "to furnish visiting nurses to those otherwise unable to secure skilled attendance in time of sickness, to teach cleanliness and proper care of the sick."[21] At the end of the first year a nurse was employed to direct the service and to supervise the nurses.

In this period it was becoming increasingly popular for persons interested in charitable and philanthropic work to band together and form settlements or settlement houses in the slums of the larger cities. Some of the groups were sponsored by universities, and graduate students and their wives lived in the settlement houses which became the base of their operations. Others were composed of groups of men and women who were concerned about the plight of the poor and felt they could contribute most to understanding and alleviating some of their miseries by living among the people and becoming intimately involved in their everyday problems. Activities and programs of all kinds were developed in the settlement houses to meet the needs of the people in the neighborhoods in which the houses were established. Many of the leaders in the settlement house movement became very active in bringing to the attention of the public the miserable conditions of the lives of the poor, and took leadership in agitating for social legislation to change conditions.

In 1893 Lillian Wald and her friend Mary Brewster, both trained nurses and wealthy in their own right, launched the district nursing service for the sick poor in New York. They moved into the neighborhood because they felt they would be more readily available to the people and would be looked upon as friends and neighbors. They became interested in all aspects of the community and were instrumental in establishing the Henry Street Settlement House. Its program included many activities for the people in the community; however, nursing always remained one of the major activities. From the inception of the nursing program the nurses were not identified with any one physician, with a free dispensary, or with a religious group. The patients were always charged fees according to their ability to pay. Calls were received from all physicians as well as from the people themselves, and the nurses maintained strict professional relationships with the physicians and the patients. Many of these ideas were revolutionary and laid the basis for a whole new relationship between the patient and the nurse. From the beginning nursing was under the supervision of nurses. Lillian Wald also believed that nursing should be aligned with the official health agency, and made arrangements with the health department for the nurses to wear an insignia which signified they were under the auspices of the board of health.

It was Lillian Wald who first used the term *public health nurse*, and she described her reason as follows:

> We called our enterprise "public health nursing." Our basic idea was that the nurse's peculiar introduction to the patient and her organic relationship with the neighborhood should constitute the starting point for a universal service to the region. Our purpose was in no sense to establish an isolated undertaking. We planned to utilize, as well as to be implemented by, all agencies and groups of whatever creed which were working for social betterment, private as well as municipal. Our scheme was to be motivated by a vital sense of the interrelation of all these forces. For this reason we considered ourselves best described by the term "public health nurse."[22]

At about the same time in Los Angeles a group of women in another settlement, called the College Settlement, appealed to the City Council for a monthly allowance for the salary of a district nurse who would give nursing care to the sick poor in their homes. The City Council agreed, and in 1898 the first nurse paid for by public funds started work under the direction of the Committee of Women in the College Settlement.

By 1900, there were twenty district nursing organizations employing 200 nurses.[23] Most were in the large cities, but some were also in the smaller communities. Each developed in its own way with no uniformity in organizational structure, sponsor, methods, records, hours of work, policies, finances, or services. This approach, similar to that of other endeavors in the United States, was consistent with the philosophy of individualism that was prevalent at that time. The federal government still maintained its laissez-faire attitude and had not as yet assumed any responsibility for the overall health of the people. In contrast, in England where district nursing was also a voluntary movement, a centralized, voluntary, uniform system of organization was being developed.

In spite of the diversity of district nursing organizations in the United States, the groundwork was being laid for their further expansion and development. Some of the basic principles of public health nursing were becoming apparent. It was increasingly evident that nursing should be available to all who were sick, regardless of ability to pay or religious affiliation; a definite distinction was being made between nursing and almsgiving; nurses were beginning to recognize the importance of keeping records; professional relationships between the doctor and nurse were carefully guarded and maintained; and the importance of cooperation with other groups in the community was being stressed in order to provide the best care to the patient. It was recognized that district nurses needed more preparation than they received in hospital programs.

SUMMARY

In any society, at any point in time, there are certain pervasive ideas and beliefs which people hold as values and which strongly influence decisions which they will make about those things which affect their very way of life. Some of the overriding ideas in the post–Civil War period were:

1. America was a land of opportunity, and anything was possible.
2. Hard work was worth the effort and would pay off—if not in the present, then certainly in the future.
3. This was a free country, a haven for everyone, and the doors would be open for those who wished to enter.
4. Those whom the country had favored with good fortune should show their gratitude by helping those who were less fortunate.
5. Public education was important if a free society was to grow and prosper.
6. Higher education was important for men.
7. Women's place was in the home for the bearing and rearing of children.
8. Individualism was paramount, and the role of the government was to make individualism possible.
9. The community was not responsible for the welfare of its people.

This was a period of rapid growth and progress, and there were many people who had different dreams and ideas for this young country. Many felt that

1. Women should have more independence and freedom, a greater voice in decision making, and equal opportunity for higher education.
2. Those concerned about problems of real social import, such as unhealthy slum conditions, poor environment, and deplorable care in hospitals, should organize and do something to change the situation.

Expansion of the railroads, industrialization, developments in science and technology, improved communication, progress in education, and changes in the role of women challenged many of the generally accepted beliefs of the times and influenced the ideas of many about the directions of America for the future. By the end of the period, there was:

1. More acceptance of the value of higher education for women, with increasing numbers of women enrolled in colleges and universities.
2. More recognition of the rights of women and their potential contribution to society. Women were demonstrating leadership and organizational ability and were seeking opportunities outside of the home.
3. A growing dream that the fruits of knowledge, industrialization, science, and technology should be available to everyone. This was beginning to happen.
4. Realization that the community could do something about its problems. A reform movement which was later to grow and flourish had already begun.

The development of nursing and district nursing in this period was an inevitable outgrowth of the times and all the forces that were being generated in society. It is impossible to separate out any one of the developments as generating the most important forces as it was a combination of the total. Perhaps nursing was an idea whose time had come. The industrial revolution, which was improving the quality of life for many, was also helping to pinpoint the discrepancies between the "haves" and the "have-nots." At the same time people were learning more about the increasing plight of the poor as wave after wave of immigrants settled in the slums of cities. A social consciousness which was characterized by idealism and humanitarianism was gaining momentum among various groups of people, particularly the better-educated women. This idealism and humanitarianism was the overriding impetus contributing to the development of nursing. Nursing also had great appeal to women who were rebelling against a restrictive society which said women's place was in the home. A whole new era for women was developing, and nursing speeded this development by providing a new occupation in which women from all segments of society could participate. Caring for the sick was a tangible expression of one's humanitarianism and tended to give one a sense of satisfaction or fulfillment. The harder one worked, the more she could contribute to the easing of suffering of others. Thus, the stage was set for all kinds of exploitation of nurses. Hard work, militarylike discipline, social isolation, and little or no education other than what was learned on the job were accepted without question. The overriding mission was service to the sick, and the other factors were only tangential to that mission. Protection of the woman by the man was a pervasive theme of the times, so the domination of nursing by medicine was a natural outgrowth.

Interested citizen groups spearheaded the development of both hospital nursing and district nursing. However, as hospital nursing became more and more dominated by physicians, the role of the citizen diminished. On the other hand, the development of district nursing was contingent from the beginning on citizen participation. Citizen groups were responsible for organizing the service, for policies governing the organization, for interpreting to the community what the nurses could do—in other words, doing everything they could to make it possible for the nurse to use her knowledge and skill in taking care of the sick poor in their own homes. In many instances the citizen groups consisted of wealthy women who were seeking a way to do good, and district nursing provided this outlet. Unfortunately, this lady-bountiful attitude also carried over in their relationships with the nurses whom they employed, and this often hampered the development of a viable partnership between the nurses and the lay groups. However, the seeds were being sown, and a model of lay and professional collaboration was evolving. District nursing was also moving in different directions from hospital nursing in other areas. Because district nurses were less isolated from the people and their day-by-day problems, they soon recognized that nurses needed more education to understand these problems and how to help the people cope with them. The sick poor who lived in the slums of the larger cities were their main focus, but by the end of the period this emphasis was beginning to shift. There was some thinking that district nursing should be available to everyone. Those who could pay for the service should do so, but no one should be refused service because of inability to pay.

As was mentioned earlier, the development of nursing and district nursing during this period was inevitable. The impact of this development had far-reaching effects. Probably the most important was on the role of women and their place in society. Nursing was not only a whole new occupation for women, but it generated the development of other occupations in which women could participate.

On the other hand, the germination of nursing in the hospital with the long hours and heavy emphasis on service sapped the energy of the nurses and left them little time to think about the direction nursing should take. Thus, the apprenticeship system of education for nursing became entrenched, and the nurse as the handmaiden of the physician was generally accepted. By the end of the period, however, some nurses were challenging these assumptions, and agitation was beginning for better education and for some control of the quality of nursing practice.

REFERENCES

1. Bureau of the Census, *A Century of Population Growth: 1790–1900* (Washington, D.C.: Government Printing Office, 1909), p. 55.
2. M. B. Greenbie, *Lincoln's Daughters of Mercy* (New York: G P. Putnam's Sons, 1944), pp. 76–77.

3. *Ibid.*, p. 216.
4. W. G. Smillie, *Public Health—Its Promise for the Future* (New York: The Macmillan Company, 1955), frontispiece.
5. O. Handlin, *The Americans* (Boston: Little, Brown and Company, 1963), p. 270.
6. F. R. Dulles, *The United States Since 1865* (Ann Arbor: University of Michigan Press, 1959), p. 91.
7. A. W. Calhoun, *A Social History of the American Family,* vol. 3 (Cleveland: The Arthur E. Clark Company, 1919), p. 66.
8. Dulles, *op. cit.*, p. 90.
9. Bureau of the Census, *op. cit.*, p. 55.
10. L. M. Hacker and B. B. Kendrick, The United States Since 1865 (New York: F. S. Crofts and Company, 1935), p. 139.
11. E. A. Ross, *Changing America* (New York: The Century Company, 1919), p. 6.
12. Dulles, *op. cit.*, p. 104.
13. H. W. Hill, *The New Public Health* (New York: The Macmillan Company, 1916), p. 30.
14. N. M. Butler, ed., *Education in the United States,* vols. 1, 2 (Albany, N.Y.: J. B. Lyon Company, 1900), p. 352.
15. Dulles, *op. cit.*, p. 187.
16. H. Shyrock, *The History of Nursing* (Philadelphia: W. B. Saunders Company, 1959), p. 300.
17. M. M. Roberts, *American Nursing* (New York: The Macmillan Company, 1954), p. 25.
18. Nurses' Associated Alumnae of the United States, "Minutes of Proceedings Fifth Annual Convention, Chicago, May 1, 2, and 3, 1902," *Amer. J. Nurs.* 2 (July 1902):766.
19. M. Jacques, *District Nursing* (New York: The Macmillan Company, 1911), pp. 6–12.
20. A. M. Brainard, *Evolution of Public Health Nursing* (Philadelphia: W. B. Saunders Company, 1922), p. 207.
21. *Ibid.*, p. 219.
22. M. Wales, *The Public Health Nurse in Action* (New York: The Macmillan Company, 1941), foreword, p. xi.
23. Shyrock, *op. cit.*, p. 298.

BIBLIOGRAPHY

Allen, F. L. *The Big Change.* New York: Harper and Brothers, 1952.

American Public Health Association. *A Half Century of Public Health—Jubilee Historical Volume of the American Public Health Association.* Lynn, Mass. The Nichols Press, 1921.

Babbidge, H. D., and Rosenzweig, R. M. *The Federal Interest in Higher Education.* New York: McGraw-Hill Company, Inc., 1962.

Blum, J. M. *The Promise of America.* Cambridge, Mass.: Houghton Mifflin Company, 1966.

Brainard, A. M. *Evolution of Public Health Nursing.* Philadelphia: W. B. Saunders Company, 1922.

———*Organization of Public Health Nursing.* New York: The Macmillan Company, 1919.

Brockett, L. P. *Woman: Her Rights, Wrongs, Privileges, and Responsibilities.* Hartford: L. Stebbins, 1869.

Brockett, L. P., and Vaughan, M. C. *Woman's Work in the Civil War: A Record of Heroism, Patriotism, and Patience.* Rochester, N. Y.: Curran, 1867.

Brooks, V. W. *Three Essays on America.* New York: E. P. Dutton and Company, 1934.

Bryson, L. *Facing the Future's Risks.* New York: Harper and Brothers, 1953.

Bureau of the Census. *A Century of Population Growth: 1790–1900.* Washington, D.C.: Government Printing Office, 1909.

Butler, N. M., ed. *Education in the United States,* vols. 1 and 2. Albany, N. Y.: J. B. Lyon Company, 1900.

Calhoun, A. W. *A Social History of the American Family,* vol. 3. Cleveland: The Arthur E. Clark Company, 1919.

Dawson, C. *The Crisis of Western Education.* New York: Sheed and Ward, 1961.

DeVane, W. C. *Higher Education in Twentieth Century America.* Cambridge, Mass.: Harvard University Press, 1965.

Dock, L. *A Short History of Nursing,* 2d ed. New York: G. P. Putnam's Sons, 1925.

Dolan, J. *Goodnow's History of Nursing.* 11th ed. Philadelphia: W. B. Saunders Company, 1963.

Dowd, D. F. *Modern Economic Problems in Historical Perspective.* Boston: D. C. Heath and Company, 1962.

Dulles, F. R. *The United States Since 1865.* Ann Arbor: The University of Michigan Press, 1959.

Fraser, G. W. *An Introduction to the Study of Education.* New York: Harper and Brothers, 1951.

Gardner, M. S. *Public Health Nursing.* New York: The Macmillan Company, 1916.

Garrison, F. H. *History of Medicine.* Philadelphia: W. B. Saunders Company, 1929.

Greenbie, M. B. *Lincoln's Daughters of Mercy.* New York: G. P. Putnam's Sons, 1944.

Hacker, L. M. *The Triumph of American Capitalism.* New York: Simon and Schuster, 1940.

Hacker, L. M., and Kendrick, B. B. *The United States Since 1865.* New York: F. S. Crofts and Company, 1935.

Hamburg, D. *Principles of a Growing Economy.* New York: W. W. Norton & Company, 1961.

Handlin, O. *The Americans.* Boston: Little, Brown and Company, 1963.

——— *Chance or Destiny.* Boston: Little, Brown and Company, 1955.

——— *This Was America.* London: Oxford University Press, 1949.

Hill, H. W. *The New Public Health.* New York: The Macmillan Company, 1916.

Jacques, M. *District Nursing.* New York: The Macmillan Company. 1911.

Jamieson, E. M. *Trends in Nursing History.* Philadelphia: W. B. Saunders Company, 1960.

Kaul, A. N. *The American Vision.* New Haven: Yale University Press, 1963.

Kraus, M. *The United States to 1965,* Ann Arbor: The University of Michigan Press, 1959.

Merry, E. J., and Iris, D. I. *District Nursing.* 2d ed. London: Bailliere, Tindall and Cox, 1955.

Miyakawa, T. S. *Protestants and Pioneers.* Chicago: University of Chicago Press, 1964.

Morgan, H. W., ed. *The Gilded Age.* Syracuse: Syracuse University Press, 1963.

Nurses' Associated Alumnae of the United States. "Minutes of Proceedings Fifth Annual Convention, Chicago, May 1, 2, and 3, 1902." *Amer. J. Nurs.,* 2:745–898, July 1902.

Nutting, M. A. *A Sound Educational Economic Basis for Schools of Nursing and Other Addresses.* New York: G. P. Putnam's Sons, 1926.

——— *Education Status of Nursing.* U. S. Bureau of Education Bulletin, No. 7. Washington, D. C.: Government Printing Office, 1912.

Richards, L. *Reminiscences of Linda Richards, America's First Trained Nurse.* Boston: Whitcomb and Barrows, 1911.

Riis, J. *The Battle with the Slums.* New York: The Macmillan Company, 1902.

Robb, I. H. *Educational Standards for Nurses.* 1907.

Roberts, M. M. *American Nursing.* New York: The Macmillan Company, 1954.

Ross, E. A. *Changing America.* New York: The Century Company, 1919.

Shyrock, R. H. *The History of Nursing.* Philadelphia: W. B. Saunders Company, 1959.

Smillie, W. G. *Public Health—Its Promise for the Future.* New York: The Macmillan Company, 1955.

Smillie, W. G., and Kilbourne, E. D. *Preventive Medicine and Public Health.* New York: The Macmillan Company, 1963.

Thomson, W. G. *Training Schools for Nurses.* New York: G. P. Putnam's Sons, 1883.

Wald, L. D. *Windows on Henry Street.* Boston: Little, Brown and Company, 1954.

———*The House on Henry Street.* New York: Henry Holt and Company, 1938.

Wales, M. *The Public Health Nurse in Action.* New York: The Macmillan Company, 1941.

Weeks-Shaw, C. A. *Text Book of Nursing.* New York: D. Appleton and Company, 1902.

Winslow, C.-E. A., Smillie, W. G., Doull, J. A., and Gordon, J. E. In F. H. Top, ed., *The History of American Epidemiology*. St. Louis: The C. V. Mosby Company, 1952.

Woods, R. A. *The Poor in Great Cities—Their Problems and What is Going to Solve Them*. New York: Charles Scribner's Sons, 1895.

Worcester, A. *Nurses For Our Neighbors*. Boston: Houghton Mifflin Company, 1914.

CHAPTER 2

THE PERIOD FROM 1900 TO THE NEW DEAL

OVERVIEW

By the turn of the century America was a young united nation endowed with the necessary ingredients for rapid growth and development. During the next 35 years there was phenomenal expansion in transportation, industrialization, and public education. It was a period in which nursing grew in stature, became a respected occupation for women, and demonstrated its real potential for professionalism. It was a time of study, experimentation, and evaluation, and of concern for quality of both nursing practice and education. Preparation of some nurses within institutions of higher education became a reality, made possible by the quality of leadership in nursing and the interest and support of foundations and philanthropists. The concept of the responsibility of the community for the health of its citizens became an accepted part of public health. The time was right for the phenomenal growth of public health nursing.

Social consciousness invaded every aspect of life. Voluntary agencies proliferated. The first part of the century was marked by feverish activity for social and legislative reform that would benefit all the people, instead of just a privileged few. This activity came to a halt at the time of the First World War. During the twenties people became preoccupied with enjoying the good things of life, and the prewar reform spirit was not revitalized. The end of the period was marked by a great depression which had immeasurable influence on all Americans and their way of life. It sounded the death knell to rugged individualism, proved that voluntary organizations were no longer able to meet the overwhelming social and health needs of the people, and made it imperative that the government assume its constitutional responsibility for the general welfare.

TRANSPORTATION

The automobile was to this period what the railroad had been to the preceding one. In 1900 there were only 13,824 cars in the United States.[1] They were considered status symbols which only the wealthy could afford. This was true, at least until 1908 when Henry Ford developed the Model-T and brought automobile ownership within the reach of everyone. In 1914 he introduced the assembly line in the production of his car. This method of mass production was destined to revolutionize transportation and the entire character of American society. The basis of the assembly line was that mass production of cars would lower the cost of each one and reduce the price to the buyer. The profit on an individual car would be small, but because of the larger number sold, the total profit would be large. In order for the assembly line to function successfully, each worker had to become competent in only one small phase of the total production process. By 1915 there were more than 2,225,000 registered automobiles,[2] and they were well on the way to becoming a necessity for the modern way of life.

After the war the automobile was no longer considered a luxury but an indispensable part of life. The Model-T became a symbol of democracy in which everyone could afford to own a car, thus reducing the social distance between the upper- and lower-income groups. Paved roads and highways increased and were spurred by the Federal Highways Act of 1921, which gave money to the states on a matching basis for the construction of certain highways. Filling stations and garages became commonplace. The isolation of the farmer ended, and dependence on the railroads lessened. Provincialism decreased as people traveled from one section of the country to another. Tourist homes, camp grounds, and hot dog stands mushroomed along well-traveled highways. Many people moved to the suburbs and commuted to work. Traffic congestion and parking problems grew. Automobile accidents increased in proportion to car ownership. In contrast to the pessimistic reaction to the appearance of the automobile, President Hoover's Committee on Social Trends reported "that no invention of such far-reaching importance was ever diffused with such rapidity, or so quickly exerted influence that ramified through the normal culture, transforming even habits of thought and language."[3]

By 1935, the number had risen to 3,273,874 passenger cars, and

697,367 trucks and buses for a total of 3,971,241.[4] The railroads were beginning to feel the bite of competition.

Air travel developed slowly and did not reach maturity until after 1935. The Wright brothers, in 1903, had carried out the first successful experiment with the airplane, but this event went almost unnoticed. It was not until after World War I that aviation became a commercial venture and was subsidized by the government for mail service. Delivery of mail by air was as important to this period as it was by continental railroad in 1869. By 1934 aviation had expanded with 24 American airlines carrying one-half million passengers over 51,000 miles of established air routes.[5]

INDUSTRIALIZATION AND TECHNOLOGY

At the beginning of the century industry had become big business and giant corporations, monopolies, and trusts were dominating the economy. The laissez-faire attitude of the government as well as some of the decisions of the Supreme Court favored the practices of the industrial giants. Several states had passed legislation in an attempt to exert some control but, as had happened similarly in the earlier period with the development of railroad companies, the state laws were geared to the interests of the individual states and often were unrelated to the overall needs of the country. However, the general public was becoming more aware of the effect of the practices of big business on the country as a whole and was beginning to rebel and to agitate for stronger government control in the interest of the general welfare. The government was forced to come to grips with some of the hard-core problems of industrialization, and in 1914 passed the Clayton Act, which attempted to regulate monopolistic practices and to protect the individual consumer.

Unionization of labor was gaining momentum, but there was no unified movement and only token support by the government. Some gains were being made in specialized areas, but for the most part poor working conditions, low pay, long hours of work, and the employment of women and children prevailed. The reform spirit, so prevalent in the first part of the century, had embraced the plight of workers and had been instrumental in the passage of some state legislation which favored them. However, some of these laws were declared unconstitutional by the Supreme Court. The most revolutionary change in favor of the workers was made by Henry Ford when in 1914 he shocked the world by raising the wages from $2.50 for a 9-hour day to $5.00 for an 8-hour day. At the same time the price of his car went down from $950.00 in 1909 to $290.00 in 1924.[6]

After the war the technical know-how and the ingenuity of the American people, plus the assembly-line principle of mass production, fed the healthy and growing industrial system, and the economy flourished. All sorts of consumer goods, appliances, and gadgets appeared on the market and were available to everyone in all walks of life. The acquisition of the same products by people of different socioeconomic levels tended to blur the sharp lines of distinction between the rich and the poor and to stabilize and universalize the culture.

The expansion of the movies and the radio also contributed to a more common culture. Moving pictures, which had been developed prior to the war, became a major industry in the twenties and a power for influencing public opinion. The impact of the movies was incalculable—they were the major source of entertainment and of ideas about life in general. Movie stars became the leaders, opinion makers, and pacesetters in society. The fashions, manners, morals, and ways of living depicted in the movies exerted their influence in every walk of life.

POPULATION AND IMMIGRATION

The population in 1900 was 75.9 million and the life expectancy at birth about 50 years. Within the next 25 years the population had increased to approximately 114 million, and life expectancy at birth had risen to 60 years for women and about 58 for men.[7]

Immigrants continued to pour into the country, with approximately one million admitted each year from 1900 through 1915. The earlier immigrants, who had come predominantly from the British Isles and northern Europe, had participated in the development of a young, growing country. After 1900 the immigrants came increasingly from countries of eastern and southern Europe. Because of their differing customs and traditions, they were looked down upon by the earlier arrivals, who considered them only one notch above the Negro on the social scale and invariably relegated them to menial, unskilled tasks. These immigrants were becoming an increasing threat to "purist" Anglo-Saxon Americans, and concern was rising about the pollution of native American stock. They were blamed for many evils of the times, such as increased crime and delinquency, slum conditions, prostitution, poor citizenship, and depression of wages. Unrest grew until the government was forced to do something about limiting immigration. In 1917 a literacy test was made a requirement for admission into the country but was ineffective in controlling immigration. In 1924 the National Origins Act was passed limiting the number of immigrants to 150,000 per year and setting up a quota system based upon the proportion of immigrants from each country who were here in 1920. This act sounded the death knell to immigration.

EDUCATION

An increasing desire to democratize and provide free education for all who were able to profit by it continued to permeate the American experience. Public education expanded, and by 1930 nearly all states had passed laws making education compulsory through age 16. High schools, which had geared their programs primarily for those preparing for college, were increasingly attended by students from all walks of life. By 1930 there were 3.5 million students enrolled in high school.[8] Curricula were no longer meeting the needs of the majority, and there was agitation for change. Courses in manual training, home economics, typewriting, agriculture, and vocational education appeared.

Americans are a practical people, and their fundamental instinct toward preparation for service was strong and instrumental in shaping one of the biggest innovations after 1900—the junior college. This new kind of program answered the needs of a growing industry and expanding technology. Business leaders influenced its development. There were new demands for training at the technical and semiprofessional levels. New occupations, such as engineering assistants and junior accountants, were opening up, and a new kind of initial preparation was needed. Before the war, with few exceptions, the junior college was accepted primarily as offering the first 2 years of a 4-year academic program. After the war there was a trend toward adding terminal and semiprofessional programs. In 1900 there were eight private junior colleges each with 100 or more students, and by 1934 there were 521 junior colleges. Of these, 302 were private and 219 public with a total enrollment of 107,807.[9]

Higher education in this part of the twentieth century was marked by curriculum exploration and experimentation, rapid expansion, growing student enrollment, and an increasing trend toward coeducation. Continuing attempts were made to clarify and redefine the aims and objectives of higher education in American society. There was a yearning for stability and a necessity for change. During the first 20 years of the new century educational programs were subjected to serious scrutiny, and repeated attempts were made to develop a curriculum more relevant to contemporary society. There was experimentation with curriculum design and methods of teaching. A system of free electives soon gave way to one of group requirements. New breadth of knowledge was included, and general education developed.

Continuous remodeling of the curriculum slackened in the twenties. Universities had reached maturity. State universities had begun their growth toward the gigantic institutions they were to become. A new relationship was developing between the federal government and higher education. The university had accepted its responsibility for the advancement of knowledge and for the preparation of its graduates to meet the needs of the country.

In the twenties the scientific approach had become accepted as basic to progress, and industrialists were beginning, more and more, to recognize the value of science in the development of technology. It was about this time that large-scale industrialists, whose products were based on scientific knowledge, set up their own laboratories for industrial research. Thus, they were assured that new and improved products and methods of production would be developed by means of technology.

Professional schools and graduate programs emphasizing specialization expanded and improved. The federal government was turning more and more to institutions of higher learning in meeting national needs. The findings and recommendations of the Flexner Study of Medical Schools, supported by the Rockefeller Foundation in 1910, had a profound effect on the quality of medical education as well as that of other professions.

In contrast to other countries, higher education in America developed without any centralized plan or governmental authority. Thus, it was characterized by the variety of its colleges and universities—public and private, large and small, men's and women's—and also by the diversity of its programs and offerings.

Women's colleges continued to increase in the early part of the century. They still used the model of men's colleges, which emphasized classical and scholarly activities. They tended to ignore the needs of the country and the contribution that educated women could make toward meeting these needs. It was during this time that the home economics movement began, stimulated by the passage, in 1914, of the Smith-Lever Act, which extended education in agriculture and home economics. The women leaders in this movement were service-oriented rather than reform-oriented and emphasized science rather than the humanities. There were no models available to them such as had been the case in the development of women's colleges. Consequently, institutes, departments, and colleges of home economics appeared in the land-grant colleges whose purpose was to use the knowledge of the laboratory to benefit the people. The home economics programs, similar to those in nursing, were practical and applied, with emphasis on bringing knowledge of sewing and cooking to the people. It was not until after 1920 that the scientific, educational, psychologic, and sociologic principles underlying the practical aspects were considered and that curricula designed to include both theory and practice appeared.

Women's colleges reached their peak about 1920. By this time women accounted for almost half of all college students. As college education became accepted as basic to success for both men and women, the glamour of being an educated woman began to fade and the percentage of women attending college started to decline. After 1930 women increasingly attended coeducational institutions, and no new women's colleges were founded.

WOMEN

After 1900 the role of women continued to expand. The fight for women's suffrage reached gigantic proportions, and many women were personally involved. The Prohibition movement also involved a large number of women, and their efforts had a great deal to do with the enactment by Congress in 1920 of the Volstead Act. This act prohibited the sale, manufacture, or transportation of all intoxicating beverages throughout the country. Through their crusade efforts, women became increasingly knowledgeable about the intricacies of the governmental process. After suffrage was granted some used their new knowledge in pursuing political careers.

More and more women worked in the offices of business and industrial firms. The earlier transition from sewing in the home to making garments in the factory was paralleled by the movement from home management to business endeavors. By the beginning of the war women had virtually conquered the stenographic field.

College women were entering many of the professions, and new opportunities were becoming available almost daily. The role of the wife and mother in the family was changing. Some college women were choosing careers instead of marriage, and there was much discussion about whether women could pursue both marriage and a career—this controversy is still going on today.

During World War I women were mobilized for the war effort by the Women's Committee of National Defense set up by President Wilson. Opportunities were opened up to them on a scale never before conceived possible. Millions replaced men who had left their jobs and, as during the Civil War, proved they could do the work equally well, if not better. By the end of the war women were firmly entrenched in many jobs that had previously been open only to men. The census in 1920 listed 572 occupations; of these, women were actively engaged in 537.[10] By 1930 one quarter of all women 16 years of age and over were in the labor force.[11]

After the war, with the passage of the Equal Suffrage Act, much of the militancy of women subsided. They were enjoying the fruits of the booming economy and their new-found freedom, and the Flapper era took over. A revolution occurred in women's fashions. A flat-chested figure and short skirts with long waists became the approved mode of the day. Women bobbed their hair, smoked cigarettes, drove cars, invaded speakeasies, and participated in athletics. They flaunted their sexiness and at the same time belittled the differences between the sexes. There was a whole new relationship between men and women as they participated together in work and play. More and more women attended coeducational institutions, and the decline of women's colleges began.

The Flapper era came to a close by 1930. This era, though short, gave added impetus to the emancipation of women and dispelled forever the ideal of the frail, genteel gentlewoman.

SOCIAL CONSCIOUSNESS

The period between 1900 and the First World War saw a tremendous awakening of social consciousness and is referred to as the "Age of Reform." There were many reasons for this, such as the exposure of corruption in big business and at all levels of government through articles in popular magazines which were read on a mass basis. Theodore Roosevelt referred to the writers of these artices as "muckrakers." There was increasing concern about the need for legislation for the benefit of all. The overall level of education had improved, and people in general were more aware of current conditions and problems. The gap between the rich and the poor was widening, and an upper class, with more leisure, was growing. The first generation of college women wanted to prove the value of higher education for women by doing something to help others who were less fortunate. Most important, perhaps, was the general feeling that society rather than the individual was responsible for the conditions under which people lived; therefore, society had a responsibility to change the conditions. The awakening was a mass movement, and no facet of life escaped the concern of the reformers. Individuals and groups became interested in a cause and then devoted all their energies to that one specific area of interest irrespective of the overall needs of the people. There was no unity or coordination of effort, and there were many gaps and much duplication.

The settlement house was at its heyday during the early part of the period and took the lead in agitating for social action. Settlement workers lived and worked in the slums, attempting in many ways to alleviate the miseries of the people. They took leadership through working on committees, persuading government officials, and organizing protest demonstrations and marches—all in the name of social justice. They concerned themselves with such things as housing, working conditions, hours of work for women, child labor, and health. Their efforts contributed to the assumption of responsibility by the individual states for public health, safety, and morals. Their efforts led directly to the establishment by the federal government in 1912 of the Children's Bureau, with its emphasis on the working conditions of women and children. This was the first social legislation enacted by the federal government.

Others approached reform through interest in special diseases, such as tuberculosis and cancer; problems relating to specific organs, such as blindness or deafness; special groups, such as children and pregnant women; or special phases, such as safety and planned parenthood. Voluntary organizations concerned with these and many other conditions mushroomed. They pioneered and brought their specific problems to the attention of the people. Many which started at the local and state level became national organizations. The whole voluntary public health nursing movement developed at this time.

Large foundations for specific purposes were established by the wealthy industrialists who had previously made contributions to charity. The Carnegie Foundation, the first, was concerned with the diffusion of knowledge. Others soon followed, such as the Rockefeller Foundation with its concern with the well-being of all mankind, the Commonwealth Fund with its interest in child health projects, and the Rosenwald Foundation for Negro education and medical and hospital services. By 1930 there were some 150 foundations with a combined capitalization of one billion dollars.[12]

The reform period was short-lived and terminated with World War I. Its accomplishments, however, were inestimable. It awakened the federal government to its responsibility for social welfare and demonstrated the pioneering and complementary function of the whole voluntary system within the nation.

After the war there was a marked change in the character of social consciousness in America. Emphasis shifted from attempting to change the social and economic ills of society to helping the individual remedy some of his own maladjustments. The idealism of the reform movement had been shattered by the war and its aftermath, and especially by failure of the United States to join the League of Nations. The people were preoccupied with acquiring and enjoying the fruits of a booming economy and rejected restrictions of any kind. Those who criticized existing conditions were thought to be un-American. The rugged individualism and hands-off policy of the government, so characteristic of the eighties and nineties, reappeared. The reluctance of the federal government to take any responsibility for social welfare set the stage for voluntary organizations to flourish.

As voluntary organizations proliferated, the need for financial security, coordination of activities, and equalization of monies became a necessity. The first community chest for this purpose was organized in Cleveland in 1914. By 1931 organized charity was the third largest industry in the United States, and there were almost 400 community chests spending as much as 100 million dollars per year.[13] In spite of this growth there were many gaps in meeting the economic, social, and health needs of the people. These gaps did not become apparent until the depression years.

THE DEPRESSION

So life went on in America during the 1920s. Even toward the end of the decade there was an air of optimism and a feeling of prosperity throughout the land. Economists, supposed to have their fingers on the pulse of the nation, were undisturbed. On September 3, 1929, the Dow Jones average of stock market made its famous "all-time" high. On November 13 the stock market crashed, and prices reached their lowest point. Allen vividly described its impact:

> The disaster which had taken place may be summed up in a single statistic. In a few short weeks it had blown into thin air *thirty billion dollars,* a sum almost as great as the entire cost to the United States of its participation in the World War, and nearly twice as great as the entire national debt.[14]

As the initial shock of the crash dulled, people faced the realities of a growing depression. The depression of the thirties was without parallel in the history of the country and the world. The entire economy slowed down. Business, construction, farming, mining—all were affected. Incomes decreased and markets contracted. Unemployment rose steadily. In 1931 the banks began to close, adding to the apprehension and misery. Nineteen thirty-two and 1933 were the cruelest years of all: almost one-fourth of the labor force was idle; the streets were less crowded; shops were untenanted; the breadlines were longer; and beggars increasingly apparent. Railroad trains were shorter, and only people who could afford gasoline used their own cars.

The effects of the Depression on the individual varied depending upon his age and station in life. Older people lost their jobs, often permanently. High schools had greater attendance than ever before as students were unable to find work. College graduates who were financially able preferred to go to graduate school rather than to remain idle. Hundreds of thousands of the young people who wanted to get married could not afford to. Those in the upper-income brackets took cuts in salaries and either dismissed their servants or allowed them to live in without pay. Many in the middle-income brackets, thrown out of work by contracting business, were forced to do all sorts of menial and poorly paid jobs in order to feed their families. Many had to go on relief for the first time in their lives. The hardest hit of all were the poor. Numerous writers have vividly described the misery of hundreds of homeless living in tin and tarpaper shacks, the despair of those waiting for hours in breadlines, and the tragedy of men fighting like animals over garbage in the streets. New York City Health Department reported in October 1932 that over one-fifth of the pupils in the public schools were suffering from malnutrition. Hundreds of people went without medical care, and doctors felt themselves lucky when a patient paid a bill.

Relief agencies of all kinds proliferated and tried desperately to meet overwhelming demands. The resources of private organizations were not adequate for this task. People turned more and more to Washington for leadership. Maintenance of general prosperity was not regarded as governmental responsibility. President Hoover was against the government's providing direct relief and injecting itself into business. He saw himself as the watchdog of rugged individualism. As the Depression deepened, so did dissatisfaction with the government and the country in general.

NURSING

Although nursing was an accepted and respectable occupation for women by 1900, it was still a fledgling profession and ill equipped for the turmoil ahead. During the next three decades it became intimately involved in and affected by the whole social upheaval with its reform movement, the First World War, and the Depression. Nursing was sustained, however, by its idealism and humanitarianism. Throughout these difficult times it studied, evaluated, and improved its preparation and performance; developed organizations for more effective functioning; and took definite steps toward the development of educational programs within institutions of higher education for some of its members.

By the turn of the century the demand for nurses was growing. More medical care was being given in hospitals, which were becoming more accepted for the care of the sick and were desperate for personnel. Large, small, special, and general hospitals established training schools for nurses at a phenomenal rate with utter disregard for the educational needs of the pupils. The number of schools grew from 452 in 1900 to 1,755 in 1920.[15] A few of these were good but the great majority unbelievably poor. Pupils were a source of cheap labor for the hospitals. They worked long hours and carried the main responsibility for the care of patients, with little or no supervision. Some pupils became a source of direct income and even profit to the hospitals. They were often sent out, during the early part of their training, to care for private patients in their own homes. Considerable fees were charged for this service. Adelaide Nutting reported in 1912:

> Out of the entire 692 hospitals from which statistics were recently received, 248 were found sending out their pupils into families in the community for private nursing, for periods ranging from 2 to 26 weeks, the payment for this service in almost all instances going directly to the hospital.[16]

Many graduates of the poor schools were an embarrassment to nursing at a time when the public was demanding better care. It soon became evident that some legal control was necessary to improve and maintain nursing standards. Groups of nurses in each state began to agitate for legislation to control the education of nurses and the practice of nursing. This was the first real effort of nurses as a group to influence legislation. They soon found out, as had the crusaders for women's suffrage, that they needed to know a great deal more about the legislative process. They persevered, and as a result the first state license law was passed in North Carolina in 1903. By 1913 over 20 states had legislation governing the practice of nursing and the education of nurses.[17]

Within the chaos in nursing education was a group that felt strongly that nurses should be educated in universities, similar to other professionals. The majority of colleges and universities, however, still offered classical curricula. Nursing, similar to home economics, which developed at about this time, was service oriented and did not fit into the existing pattern of higher education. The first program for the basic preparation of nurses associated with a university was inaugurated at the University of Minnesota in 1909. About this time there was also some movement toward hospital schools of nursing affiliating with institutions of higher learning. Several hospital schools had collaborative arrangements with colleges and technical schools for science courses and the use of laboratories for their pupils. College and university courses for graduate nurses were being developed. Teachers College took the lead in this. Pupils were beginning to be referred to as students for the first time. High school graduation was a requirement for entrance to several of the leading schools of nursing, and definite efforts were being made by a few to attract college graduates. Slowly progress was being made. Reform in other areas made it easier to bring about improvements in working conditions and shorter hours of work for both pupil and graduate nurses.

Recruitment of adequate numbers of suitable applicants was becoming increasingly difficult. More and more able women were going to college and paying full tuition for 4 years of education in spite of the fact that education for nursing was generally free and only 2 or 3 years in length. There were all kinds of opportunities for women. Everyone seemed to be clamoring for applicants—for teachers, for doctors, for clerical workers, and others. Recruitment problems were not peculiar to nursing. Nursing's problem, however, was particularly acute because unlike the other professions which had established themselves on an educationally sound basis, nursing was getting more and more entrenched in the apprenticeship system, which was inadequate for the needs of the growing profession.

The nursing organizations recognized their responsibility for professional leadership and looked again at their purposes and objectives. In 1911 the Nurses' Associated Alumnae became the American Nurses' Association. By 1912 public health nurses recognized the need for an organization concerned with their particular interests, and the National Organization for Public Health Nursing was started. According to Mary Gardner,

> The object of this organization shall be to stimulate responsibility for the health of the community by establishment and extension of public health nursing; to facilitate efficient cooperation between nurses, physicians, boards of trustees, and other persons interested in public health measures; to develop standards and techniques in public health nursing service; to establish a central bureau for information, reference, and assistance in matters pertaining to such services; and to publish periodicals or issue bulletins from time to time on the accomplishment of the general purposes of this organization.[18]

The National Organization for Public Health Nursing specifically differed from the other two national nursing organizations. One of the differences was that membership was open to public health nurses, public health nursing agencies, and interested citizens. One of its strengths from the beginning was in developing cooperative relationships with other health and social agencies.

The same year the American Society of Superintendents of Training Schools for Nurses became the National League for Nursing Education. It appointed an Education Committee which was specifically concerned with the problems of nursing education and the need for greater standardization and uniformity of the educational programs. *The Standard Curriculum for Nursing Schools,* the first tangible step toward improving nursing education, appeared in 1917, and had real impact at this time. It established the National League for Nursing Education as the authoritative source for information concerning nursing education.

The influence of World War I on nursing was both immediate and far-reaching. It resulted in increasing knowledge and concern on the part of the general public, including many college-trained women, about the whole system of nursing education and its weaknesses. Colleges and universities looked at nursing more seriously as a profession "here to stay." It awakened nurses themselves to the inadequacies of nursing education and laid the groundwork for the studies and changes which followed the war.

Recruitment of nurses for the army and the civilian population had immediate priority. Under the leadership of Adelaide Nutting a National Emergency Committee on Nursing was organized. It soon became the Committee on Nursing of the General Medical Board of the Council of National Defense—a committee established by President Wilson. Adelaide Nutting became the chairman and Ella Phillips Crandall the secretary of the Committee on Nursing. The plan of this committee for supplying a steady flow of nurses included a well-organized, widespread student recruitment program which resulted in increased numbers of students and a Student Nurse Reserve of many thousands. Isabel Stewart relates that

> The cooperation of public-spirited citizens was also stimulated by the close association of nursing and other groups concerned with national defense. This was true especially of the large and influential Women's Committee under Dr. Anna Howard Shaw of suffrage fame, which with its 12,000 state and local branches took over the chief responsibility for filling the Student Nurse Reserve.[19]

The shortage of nurses in hospitals during the war was eased as the student recruitment program got under way. In addition, many hundreds of women volunteered as aides. These were usually well-educated women who wanted to be of service and knew they were not prepared to be nurses.

In addition to the Committee on Nursing, there were two other committees of the Council of National Defense concerned with nursing—the Subcommittee on Public Health Nurses, with Mary Beard as chairman, and the Subcommittee on Hospitals. The problems of coordination between these subcommittees were complex and difficult. Both Ella Crandall and Mary Beard enlisted the services of the American Red Cross. The demand for public health nurses both at home and abroad was increasing. The Red Cross was asked to establish a special roster of public health nurses, who were considered war workers. Their patriotic duty was recognized by the Red Cross, which issued a special chevron for them to wear. There was a special need for public health nurses in the areas around the military cantonment areas. Mary Lent was loaned by the National Organization for Public Health Nursing to the United States Public Health Service to cooperate with the local and state agencies and develop a public health nursing program for the cantonment areas. This was the first public health nursing service to be established within the federal government.

A concerted attempt to attract some of the college women into nursing became part of the recruitment program. Letters were sent to all the women's and coeducational colleges in the country, as well as to many graduates, to determine their interest in pursuing nursing as a career. In the summer of 1918 the Vassar Training Camp was set up for college graduates and offered them a preparatory course with the assurance that it would shorten the length of training for nursing. Over 418 attended, and about one-third of these later graduated from schools of nursing and assumed leadership roles in nursing.

Currents set in motion by the war continued after the armistice. A better-informed public became increasingly concerned about the health of the people and the supply and preparation of nurses to meet the growing demands of society. Public health nursing services expanded rapidly. As the need for adequate personnel increased, so did questions about the function and preparation of the public health nurse. The Rockefeller Foundation, which had previously given financial assistance to the National Organization for Public Health Nursing, set up a conference for the consideration of some of these questions. In 1918 C-E. A. Winslow was appointed chairman of the committee to study the whole problem of public health nursing education. It soon became evident that any study of this kind must include nursing and nursing education. The committee was broadened and renamed the Committee for the Study of Nursing Education. Josephine Goldmark was appointed director of the study, which extended over a period of 3 years. Some of the recommendations of this study were:

> The quality of applicants and programs of nursing education should be strengthened and improved generally; schools of nursing should work toward increased educational and financial independence; the course should be shortened from three years to twenty-eight months by the elimination of non-educational and repetitive services; subsidiary workers should be prepared and licensed for the care of certain less critically ill patients; emphasis should be placed on special preparation, beyond the basic nursing course, for administrators and teachers for schools of nursing and for public health nurses; the university schools of nursing should be further developed and strengthened.[20]

There were two important and immediate results of this last recommendation: the founding in 1923 of both the Yale University School of Nursing, financed by the Rockefeller Foundation, and the Frances Payne Bolton School of Nursing at Western Reserve University, financed by

Frances Payne Bolton. Miss Bolton was a wealthy and influential citizen who became very much interested in University education for nurses as a result of the Goldmark Report.

The period of the twenties was one of turmoil, reevaluation, and experimentation. Schools of nursing proliferated. Prospective nursing students, recruitment personnel, nurses, and nurse educators wanted and needed more specific and definitive information about the entire nursing situation. In 1925 a program for grading schools of nursing was approved by the three national nursing organizations, and a year later the Committee on the Grading of Nursing Schools came into being. It was composed of 21 members—14 of whom represented national organizations interested in the quality and availability of nursing. The Committee undertook three major projects: a study of the supply and demand for nursing service, a job analysis of nurses, and the grading of nursing schools. Grading of schools was accomplished in 1929 and repeated in 1932. As a result several hundred of the poorer schools closed their doors, and many others improved their educational programs.

Although early connections between schools of nursing and institutions of higher education were sporadic and without uniformity, nursing schools continued to multiply. By 1931 there were 67 schools of nursing with some kind of college or university relationship, 12 percent of these being affiliated with junior colleges.[21] At the same time college education for graduate nurses was becoming more available. These developments in nursing education brought with them a whole new set of perplexing problems relating to organization, administration, financing, curriculum, and faculty and student qualifications. A series of conferences was held to discuss these problems, and there was a consensus that the advantages in these new relationships outweighed the disadvantages. The Committees on University Schools of the National League for Nursing Education took the leadership in these deliberations and continued to study the situation. In 1933 the Association of Collegiate Schools of Nursing was formed with the following purposes:

> To develop nursing education on a professional and collegiate level, to promote and strengthen relationships between schools of nursing and institutions of higher education, and to promote a study and experimentation in nursing service and nursing education.[22]

Most of the energies of the leaders in nursing during the period following the war were directed toward studying and improving the educational preparation of nurses. A few postgraduate courses were becoming available in colleges and universities for the preparation of head nurses. Graduate nurses were assuming head nurse positions in hospitals. Postgraduate courses were also available for the preparation of teachers, supervisors, and administrators in nursing. Some hospitals were developing courses for nurses who wished further clinical knowledge in special areas such as pediatrics, maternity, and the operating room. With the exception of public health nursing, universities did not accept any responsibility for the preparation of nurses for the practice of nursing. The first grading study showed that even at the very height of national prosperity many private duty nurses were unemployed. There were far more nurses than could be employed under existing conditions. On the other hand, there were too few nurses qualified for positions demanding special knowledge and skills.

By the end of the twenties the deepening depression was affecting all aspects of the American economy, and unemployment among graduate nurses was becoming pronounced. They did not escape the weary round of job hunting, reduced salaries, depleted savings, or even the bread lines. Many of the hospitals which had discontinued their schools of nursing employed graduate nurses for the first time. The numbers employed increased with the severity of the depression. Many graduates were willing to work for low salaries and even to give free service in exchange for room and board. The outcome of this was positive. Hospital administrators realized that graduate nurses gave better care to patients than did students, and a whole new area of service opened up for graduate nurses. New possibilities for the development of more independence for schools of nursing loomed on the horizon.

Nursing withstood the stresses and strains of the first three decades of the twentieth century and matured in the process. Recognition of the necessity for better education for nurses resulted in considerable improvement in nursing programs within hospitals. In addition, the foundation for future developments in collegiate education for nurses was firmly laid.

PUBLIC HEALTH NURSING

Public health nursing really came into its own during the first three decades of the twentieth century. It clarified its purposes, preparation, and organization. By 1900 the germ theory of the cause of disease was well established. Public health endeavors for the most part were geared toward the application of this theory in the control and prevention of communicable disease, with major emphasis placed upon control of the environment. In spite of these efforts the incidence of communicable disease was widespread. Williams[23] has reported that between 1890 and 1910 there was more than three times the number of deaths from typhoid fever in the United States than in some of the other countries of the world. The philosophy that the government should be responsible for the health of the community had not as yet permeated the state and local health departments. The federal government was beginning to show a little interest in its responsibility for public health, and the need for more adequate statistics about people as a whole was beginning to be recognized. The Census Bureau was established in 1902 and the Death Registration Area in 1900. In 1902 Congress also passed an act which gave legal authority for the first time to the Surgeon General of the United States and Territorial Health Officers in order to promote the interest of public health.

Many of the people involved in the reform movement were concerned about the poor health situation and the need for legislation to improve the health of the people. Industrial and technologic developments had stimulated the economy of the country, and the accumulated wealth provided a means of support for community health. Voluntary health agencies concerned with a particular disease or condition proliferated. The rapid growth of these agencies was due in part to the constant threat of communicable disease, the ineffectiveness of health departments in alleviating this threat, and the widespread feeling of social consciousness with its urgency to improve the plight of the poor. The philosophy underlying the development of voluntary health agencies was that of the importance of community action in the protection of the health of the individual. This was exemplified by the interest and involvement of citizens in establishing and financing the services that were provided.

As the services offered by the voluntary health agencies expanded, so did the demand for nurses in specialized programs. The tuberculosis crusade was the first to recognize the contribution of the nurse as a teacher of hygiene and sanitation in the control of tuberculosis. The high mortality rate of infants led to the development of infant welfare stations, and more nurses were demanded to work in this specialized area. It was not long before nurses were being sought to function in specialized areas such as communicable disease, tuberculosis, venereal disease, mental health, schools, factories, and many others.

The voluntary movement in district nursing, which mushroomed after the turn of the century, was consistent with the development of other voluntary health agencies. The citizens recognized the needs for nursing care to sick people in their homes and in turn organized and contributed 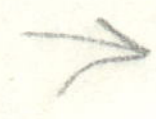 funds to meet these needs. The voluntary nursing agencies contributed by innovating new programs, demonstrating the need for public health nursing, and supplementing governmental nursing services. This was exemplified by Lillian Wald at Henry Street when she demonstrated the value of a nurse in the public schools. As a result of this experiment, the Board of Education in New York City, in 1902, employed the first school nurse in the United States. There were several leaders in nursing who thought that public health nursing should be a responsibility of government; some local health departments were employing nurses.

Public health nursing was well established by the time the reform movement in public health took place around 1910. Although the general reform movement was beginning to show some signs of waning by this time, it resulted in legislation and philosophic changes in society which strongly influenced the whole development and approach of public health. It resulted in health legislation which gave authority to the states for the protection of the individual and made the health of the individual a community responsibility. At the same time the emphasis in the control of disease was broadening to include the promotion of the health of the individual in his environment, rather than just controlling the environment. It was at this time that district nursing, which had pioneered in health promotion and disease prevention by working with people in their own homes, became a ready and able partner in the whole public health movement. According to Winslow public health nurses provided the first effective link between a planned community health program and the individual family in the home. Winslow further states that "for what the nursing profession has accomplished and for the leadership of the board member group in that accomplishment, we owe an incalculable debt of gratitude."[24] It was at this time that the functions of the district nurse expanded and more nearly met those of a public health nurse, as envisioned by Lillian Wald when she started district nursing services at Henry Street. Public health nursing services were organized in a variety of ways. They were offered by large and small visiting nurse associations, medical dispensaries, and boards of health. In some instances visiting nurse associations in the larger cities sold services to smaller surrounding communities or combined their services with boards of health or boards of education. In 1909 the Metropolitan Life Insurance Company, as a result of an experiment with Henry Street, offered nursing service to certain of its policyholders. Its plan was to affiliate with existing agencies rather than to duplicate services, and to employ its own nurses only when no other service was available. By 1928 it had affiliations with 953 organizations and employed an independent staff of 592 nurses. There was also great variation in the development of rural public health nursing services, depending on the needs and resources of individual communities. Public health nurses could be found working under many auspices—including the Red Cross.

Irrespective of the kind of arrangement, stress was laid upon organizing to meet the needs of the community, and upon the premise that each local community must determine how its service should be organized. In spite of the flexibility and diversity of the programs and agencies, some principles of administration in public health nursing were evolving. Some of these were: the need for sound financing of public health nursing; the necessity for the involvement of community people in establishing and financing the program; the recognition that the program of the agency should be based upon the needs of the community; the necessity for nursing to collaborate with other health and social agencies in the community in order to avoid gaps and duplication in service; and the importance of records and statistics as necessary tools in the development of public health nursing. At the same time the relationship of the health of the family to the health of the community was beginning to be recognized, and the family as a whole was becoming the focus for the public health nurse.

As the role and activities of the district nurse broadened and diversified, it soon became apparent that further educational preparation beyond the hospital was necessary. A few of the visiting nurse associations instituted in-service education programs for their nurses, but there were no organized programs for the preparation of district nurses. The first course for graduate nurses who wished to specialize in district nursing was established by the Instructive District Nursing Association of Boston in 1906. The course was 4 months in length and included lectures and practice. Several of the larger visiting nurse associations established similar courses in an attempt to meet the need for better-prepared district nurses. It was not until 1910, when a Department of Nursing and Health for graduate nurses was established at Teachers College, Columbia University, that institutions of higher learning assumed any responsibility for the education of public health nurses. The Department of Nursing and Health was an outgrowth of a course in hospital economics for graduate nurses established at Teachers College in 1899 and sponsored by the Society of Superintendents of Training Schools. The course had been designed to prepare women for administrative and teaching positions in hospitals but had never been satisfactorily developed because of lack of funds. A gift of $150,000 from Helen Jenkins made the Department of Nursing and Health financially stable and permanent. This was the first time that money was given to support any nursing education in the United States. Three programs of study were offered: the preparation of teachers and supervisors for training schools; the preparation of administrators of hospitals and training schools; and the preparation of public health nurses.[25]

As a result of the program at Teachers College, some of the visiting nurse associations which offered special public health nursing courses for the preparation of their own staff developed collaborative relationships with colleges and universities. For example, the course at the

Cleveland Visiting Nurse association was transferred to Western Reserve University in 1911, and the one conducted by the Instructive District Nursing Association of Boston was transferred to Simmons College in 1912. By 1921 there were 15 colleges and universities offering courses in public health nursing which met the educational standards developed by the National Organization for Public Health Nursing.[26] By 1929 the National Organization for Public Health Nursing had established a procedure for grading postgraduate courses in public health nursing, and had approved courses that met the following minimum requirements: a qualified nurse director; affiliation with a school of collegiate grade; a budget; and an academic-year program with didactic and field instruction. By this time, partly as a result of the introduction into universities of public health nursing courses, 5-year undergraduate programs in nursing were established in a few colleges and universities. Seven of the approved postgraduate public health nursing courses were connected with 5-year university programs and provided the fifth year in public health nursing to an increasing number of undergraduate nursing students.[27]

It was during the twenties that public health recognized the relationship of the health of the individual to the economic security of the community and assumed responsibility for community health. By 1920 all the states and most of the large cities had health departments which were staffed by large numbers of people. The largest proportion of professional workers were public health nurses. The importance of health education, on both an individual and a broad community-wide basis, had its beginnings during this time and was fostered by the developments in mass communication, such as the radio, moving pictures, and the increasing circulation of newspapers and magazines. In 1924 the Shephard-Towner Act was passed, which gave money to the states on a matching basis to enable each state to establish a program for the promotion of the welfare and hygiene of mothers and infants. This act, which was vigorously opposed by many as a violation of states' rights, established the pattern to be followed later by the federal government, that of awarding monies on a matching basis to the states for the alleviation of a vaaiety of health hazards.

Paralleling developments in public health were developments in public health nursing. Public health nursing was in its heyday during the twenties. It was the standard bearer for both the improvement and expansion of health services. It took leadership in establishing standards of nursing practice; demanded academic education for public health nurses; worked with citizens and other professionals in developing and improving services; and established a sound basis for cost and time studies. It collaborated with other professional organizations in carrying out the first real census of public health nurses, which became a model for later studies. Public health nursing became part of both state and local health departments and expanded its services in both rural and urban areas. It influenced and was in turn influenced by health and welfare legislation.

Public health nurses brought health services directly to the people and were welcomed into the homes of the rich and poor alike. They not only gave bedside nursing care but also interpreted the latest knowledge of disease prevention and health promotion. They helped to broaden the nation's concept of health. They also demonstrated that prevention of disease and promotion of health, as well as care of the sick, were a responsibility of nursing.

The family had become recognized as the unit of service for the public health nurse. At the same time, in spite of this, many agencies were employing specialists in such areas as venereal disease, tuberculosis, maternal and child health, and school nursing. There was growing recognition that specialists were needed for leadership, but also that duplication and gaps in service resulted. By the middle of the twenties the trend was toward generalization of services, through which one staff nurse, adequately supervised and supported by well-trained supervisors and consultants, gave total service to an individual family.

The first census of public health nurses in the United States as of January 1, 1924, carried out by the National Organization for Public Health Nursing, was remarkable in its organization and management. The cooperation of those participating was a real tribute to the National Organization for Public Health Nursing. It was the most comprehensive study of its kind to date and included 752 cities of populations over 10,000 as well as smaller cities and rural areas of the country. This first official census showed that there were 3,267 organizations employing 11,152 full-time graduate nurses.[28] It also revealed variation in financing, and gaps and duplication of services. Forty-seven percent of agencies were supported wholly by public funds; an additional 28 percent received some public funds; and 25 percent were supported wholly by private funds. Nursing service was entirely free in all but 24 percent of the agencies.[29]

One of the statistical problems encountered by the National Organization for Public Health Nursing in planning the census had been the lack of an actual definition of public health nursing. As a result, information about qualifications had not been included in the census. A year later, the American Public Health Association, the National Organization for Public Health Nursing, and the state and provincial health authorities formed a joint committee to consider minimal qualifications for public health nursing at the staff, supervisory, and director levels. They recommended qualifications for 1925 and projected them for 1930. It is interesting to note that two years of high school was acceptable in 1925 for all three levels, but completion of high school was a requirement by 1930. Professional, academic, and experience requirements were progressive, and the 1930 qualifications for staff nurses included theoretic and practical experience in one or more of the following: public health nursing, communicable disease nursing, tuberculosis nursing, hospital social services, or mental hygiene. Qualification for supervisors and directors required at least 2 years of public health nursing experience and a recognized public health nursing course, including theory and practice in an educational institution. College education, or at least 2 years beyond the minimal educational requirements, was considered desirable.

The next few years were tremendously important ones for public health nursing. A manual presenting general underlying principles and guidelines for public health nursing was published in 1926, and revised in 1932. The first cost studies for public health nursing were published in 1926, and increasing numbers of comparative cost figures became available for use in planning. An appraisal form was developed 2 years later and was instrumental in directing attention to both quality and quantity of service.

By the early thirties the effects of the depression were omnipresent. Public health nursing services had to be curtailed. Salaries decreased. Unemployment was on the rise. However, public health nursing was, on the whole, in a peculiarly fortunate position to withstand the depression. It had formulated its objectives and worked out a sound basis of organization. As the need for service increased, public health nursing was in a position to respond and to become more intimately involved with the community in meeting these needs.

SUMMARY

The period between 1900 and the New Deal was bisected by the First World War with all its horror, and ended with the greatest depression the country had ever known—a depression which resulted in the New Deal and a change in the whole relationship between rugged individualism and the role of the government. The challenges to previously accepted ideas and beliefs were forceful and insistent. Endemic values were changing and priorities being reordered. There was now a general feeling that

1. The doors should no longer be wide open to immigrants, who were a growing threat to Anglo-Saxonism and were held responsible by many for a large share of the ills of society.

2. Society and not the individual was responsible for poverty, and society must do something about these social ills. The need for social reform was given high priority.
3. The gap between the rich and the poor was widening. The rich must organize and contribute to help the poor.
4. Education was not only important for a free society, but was necessary for a democracy if it were to survive.
5. Americans were a practical people, and their education should be practical and relevant.
6. Higher education was as valuable for women as for men.
7. The suburbs were increasingly desirable places for middle- and upper-class families to live and raise their children.
8. Women should have equal rights and should work toward making these a reality.
9. Science, technology, and research were basic to industry, education, and progress itself.
10. There was more than one cause for environmental and disease conditions.
11. The size and composition of the American family was changing.
12. An overriding optimism prevailed, even right up to the time of the depression.

The effects of war on any country are profound and incalculable. The aftermath of World War I was no exception. The prewar frenzy for social, legislative, and educational reform died out after the war. Emphasis shifted from helping others to enjoying the good things of life—many of which had been made possible by progress in transportation, industry, and education.

The depression tested individual and voluntary effort to solve the problems of the country almost to the breaking point. The resources of private individuals and groups, no matter how dedicated, were just not adequate for the task. The results of the depression demanded that the federal government assume a whole new kind of responsibility for the general welfare. A new partnership between the government and voluntary organizations began to develop, and there was a growing realization that

1. Although individualism was still important, it might have to be submerged for the good of all the people.
2. The government not only should but must assume responsibility for the general welfare.

The idealism and humanitarianism which continued to dominate nursing during this period hampered reform in both the education and practice of nursing. Society idealized the nurse as an "angel of mercy" who soothed the feverish brows of the sick. Thus, persons who selected nursing as a career were conditioned by society's views and tended to perpetuate them. This image, with its implications for dedicated service, was to haunt nursing for many years and put a damper on the reforms necessary for the development of nursing as a scholarly profession.

At the same time, changes were occurring in society at large which pinpointed the need for better education for nurses. It was generally accepted that education was necessary for a society's survival, and public education became more readily available for everyone. Higher education became acceptable for women, and the idea that women could pursue both a career and marriage gained momentum. Graduate education expanded, professional schools developed, and research became important for progress.

Nursing was struggling to get into the mainstream of education but was having a difficult time because of an entrenched apprenticeship system which it could not shake, despite valiant efforts by a few dedicated individuals. Also, for much of the period, curricula in colleges were still oriented toward the classics, and this made it doubly difficult to conceive of nursing, which was practice-oriented, as being included in the existing structure of higher education. Other professions for women were developing, such as social work and home economics, and were faced with a similar dilemma. However, as these professions developed, men also became attracted to them. In many instances it was men who took the leadership in establishing standards for education, which were then equally applicable to the men and women in the profession. Nursing, on the other hand, was exclusively a female occupation and was under the domination of physicians. The physicians assumed leadership over the educational standards for nurses as well as those for the medical profession. Thus, the educational standards were higher for the physician, who was usually a man, and lower for the nurse, who was usually a woman. Perhaps if men had been attracted to nursing in its formative stage, the father image of the physician would not have become so strongly entrenched, and nursing would have moved more quickly into the mainstream of higher education.

The unchecked growth of hospital training schools for nurses and the lack of uniform standards for practice and education were an overriding concern of nursing during this period. Some of the thoughtful leaders in nursing realized that nursing had to get itself organized and set up its own standards if it were to develop and survive as a profession.

At the beginning of the century when the reform movement reached its zenith, there was feverish activity in all areas with no coordination of efforts or any overall master plan. It was almost as if there was a sudden reawakening of the need for reform in every area of life. The important thing was to bring about change, and it really did not matter too much who selected which endeavor. Individualism was the order of the day, and there was ample opportunity for individuals or groups to develop their special interests without government interference. Thus, it was natural for special interest groups in nursing to evolve, and the stage was set for the development of public health nursing as a separate entity.

Reform in nursing took place in relation to where nursing was practiced. Institutional nursing was greatly influenced by the hospital with its boundaries and problems, whereas public health nursing, which was practiced outside of the hospital, was more closely related to the community and the forces affecting society as a whole. With the increase in scientific knowledge and technology the hospital became more acceptable for the care of the sick, and the focus of nursing, as well as of medicine, was centered on the sick individual. Nurses needed knowledge about disease and its treatment in order to carry out the medical plan of care. Students were the primary providers of nursing care in the hospital and were ideal handmaidens to the physician. Public health nurses, on the other hand, were translating the benefits of scientific knowledge directly to the family in the home for the purpose of health promotion and disease prevention. Trained nurses were the primary providers of nursing care and were not necessarily dependent upon a medical plan of care. Team relationships with the physician and other health professionals were developing as it became more and more evident that the health needs of families could not be met by any one discipline working in isolation. The beginnings of the public health team consisting of the public health physician, the public health nurse, and the sanitarian were gaining impetus.

Tremendous energy was expended on defining educational standards for nurses, by both institutional nursing and public health nursing. The major thrust was toward establishing uniform standards for nursing education and practice. Institutional nursing recognized the need for preparing administrators and teachers in institutions of higher learning, and a few programs one year in length were established. Public health nursing at the same time was giving high priority to the need for better-educated nurses in order to provide better service to patients. One-year university programs were established with public health nursing practice as the objective. Educational standards were developed for staff nurses, supervisors, and administrators in public health nursing and were included as part of the requirements for employment under many of the Civil Service Commissions. Also, in-service education, in which the employing agency took responsibility for conducting educational programs to help nurses keep abreast of new developments in order to bring this knowledge to their patients, was reinforced. The public health nurse was becoming a familiar and welcome figure in the homes of people in all walks of life. Developments in transportation, particularly the Model-T Ford, made it possible for her to reach more people and to extend her services to rural areas. She was often the only person in smaller communities who was concerned about the health status of the community, and in many instances her endeavors led to the development of a full-time health department.

The rapid development of voluntary visiting nurse associations with strong citizen involvement speeded the development of sound personnel policies and regular working hours for public health nurses. Citizen participation in public health nursing culminated in the establishment of the National Organization for Public Health Nursing with its emphasis on lay membership. The importance of working collaboratively with other professionals in solving health problems early became one of the armamentaria of public health nurses. This was vividly demonstrated in 1923 when Public Health Nursing became a section in the American Public Health Association.

Nursing research did not take on stature until a much later time, but a research approach, the value of statistics, fact-finding, and the ordering of data were early tools of public health nursing. Time and cost studies in public health nursing were models that were used by other groups in studying costs. Collaborative relationships with other national organizations in the census of public health nurses also became a model for multidiscipline collaboration.

Public health nursing was in its heyday during this period. No endeavor was too great, and every aspect of the life of the family and the community was the territory of the public health nurse. The independent functions of nursing were demonstrated, although not identified, and a vision of nursing as a profession was created.

REFERENCES

1. L. Allen, *The Big Change* (New York: Harper & Brothers, 1952), p. 124.
2. L. D. Morris, *Not So Long Ago* (New York: Random House, 1949), p. 324.
3. *Ibid.*, p. 284.
4. J. B. Rae, *The American Automobile* (Chicago: University of Chicago Press, 1965), p. 238.
5. F. R. Dulles, *The United States Since 1865* (Ann Arbor: The University of Michigan Press, 1959), p. 311.
6. F. Mowry, *The Urban Nation 1920–1960* (New York: Hill & Wang, 1965), p. 13.
7. W. Smillie, *Public Health—Its Promise for the Future* (New York: The Macmillan Company, 1955), frontispiece.
8. L. M. Hackett and B. B. Kendrick, *The United States Since 1865* (New York: F. S. Crofts and Company, 1935), p. 691.
9. M. Brick, *Form and Focus for the Junior College Movement* (New York: Bureau of Publications, Teachers College, Columbia University, 1964), pp. 24–25.

10. L. D. Morris, *Postscript to Yesterday* (New York: Random House, 1947), p. 50.
11. L. Bryson, ed., *Facing the Future's Risks* (New York: Harper & Brothers, 1953), p. 191.
12. Hackett and Kendrick, *op. cit.*, p. 689.
13. *Ibid.*
14. F. L. Allen, *Since Yesterday: The Nineteen-Thirties in America, September 3, 1929–September 3, 1939* (New York: Harper & Brothers, 1940), p. 26.
15. E. Jamieson, F. Sewall, L. Gjertson, *Trends in Nursing History,* 2d ed. (Philadelphia: W. B. Saunders Company, 1960), p. 416.
16. M. A. Nutting, *Educational Status of Nursing,* U.S. Bureau of Education Bulletin 1912 (Washington, D.C.: Government Printing Office, 1912), p. 21.
17. I. Stewart, *The Education of Nurses* (New York: The Macmillan Company, 1950), p. 140.
18. M. S. Gardner, *Public Health Nursing* (New York: The Macmillan Company, 1916), p. 31.
19. Stewart, *op. cit.*, p. 196.
20. M. Roberts, *American Nursing* (New York: The Macmillan Company, 1954), p. 179.
21. *Proceedings of the 37th Annual Convention of the National League for Nursing Education in 1931,* p. 134.
22. Stewart, *op. cit.*, p. 231.
23. R. C. Williams, *The United States Public Health Service* (Bethesda, Md.: The Commissioned Officers Association of the United States Public Health Service, Box 5874, 1951), p. 140.
24. C.-E. A. Winslow, "Housing and Health," *The Public Health Nurse* 32 (July 1940):437.
25. Nutting, *op. cit.*, pp. 8–9.
26. A. Strong, "The Education of Public Health Nurses," *The Public Health Nurse* 13 (May 1921):226.
27. National Organization for Public Health Nursing, "Post Graduate Courses in Public Health Nursing," *The Public Health Nurse* 21 (February 1929):94.
28. ———. "Census of Public Health Nurses in the United States, January 1, 1924, "*The Public Health Nurse* 18 (January 1926):24–27.
29. M. Clark, "The Census and Public Health Nursing Traditions," *The Public Health Nurse* 18 (August 1926):464, 465, 467.

BIBLIOGRAPHY

Allen, F. L. *The Big Change.* New York: Harper and Brothers, 1952.

———. *Since Yesterday: The Nineteen-Thirties in America, September 3, 1929–September 3, 1939.* New York: Harper and Brothers, 1940.

Berelson, B. *Graduate Education in the United States.* New York: McGraw-Hill Company, 1960.

Brick, M. *Form and Focus for the Junior College Movement.* New York: Bureau of Publications, Teachers College, Columbia University, 1964.

Bryson, L., ed. *Facing the Future's Risks.* New York: Harper and Brothers, 1953.

Clark, M. "The Census and Public Health Nursing Traditions." *Amer. J. Public Health,* 29:128–34, February 1939.

Committee on the Grading of Nursing Schools. *Nursing Schools Today and Tomorrow.* New York City, 1934.

Deming, D. "Milestones of the Past Fifteen Years in Public Health Nursing." *Amer. J. Public Health,* 29:128–34, February 1939.

DeVane, W. C. *Higher Education in Twentieth Century America.* Cambridge, Mass.: Harvard University Press, 1965.

Dowd, D. *Modern Economic Problems in Historical Perspective.* Boston: D. C. Heath and Company, 1962.

Dulles, F. R. *The United States Since 1865.* Ann Arbor: The University of Michigan Press, 1959.

Gardner, M. S. *Public Health Nursing.* New York: The Macmillan Company, 1916.

Hackett, L., and Kendrick, B. *The United States Since 1865.* New York: F. S. Crofts and Company, 1935.

Jamieson, E., Sewall, F., and Gjertson, L. *Trends in Nursing History.* 2nd ed. Philadelphia: W. B. Saunders Company, 1960.

Morris, L. D. *Not So Long Ago.* New York: Random House, 1949.

———. *Postscript to Yesterday.* New York: Random House, 1947.

Mowry, F. *The Urban Nation 1920–1960.* New York: Hill and Wang, 1965.

National Organization for Public Health Nursing. "Census of Public Health Nurses in the United States—1924." *The Public Health Nurse,* 18:24–27, January 1926.

———. "Census of Public Health Nurses in the United States, January 1, 1924." *The Public Health Nurse,* 18:249–313, June 1926.

———. "Post Graduate Courses in Public Health Nursing." *The Public Health Nurse,* 21:93–95, February 1929.

———. *Principles and Practices in Public Health Nursing Including Cost Analysis.* New York: The Macmillan Company, 1932.

———. "Standardizing Qualifications for Public Health Nursing Positions," *The Public Health Nurse,* 17:297–99, June 1925.

Newcomer, M. *A Century of Higher Education for American Women.* New York: Harper and Brothers, 1959.

Nutting, M. A. *Educational Status of Nursing.* Washington, D.C.: U.S. Bureau of Education Bulletin 1912, Government Printing Office, 1912.

Petry, L. "Basic Professional Curricula in Nursing Leading to Degrees." *Amer. J. Nurs.,* 37:287–297, March 1937.

Proceedings of the 37th Annual Convention of the National League for Nursing Education in 1931.

Rae, J. B. *The American Automobile.* Chicago: University of Chicago Press, 1965.

Roberts, M. *American Nursing.* New York: The Macmillan Company, 1954.

Schlesinger, A. *Age of Roosevelt—Crisis of the Old Order 1919–1933.* Boston: Houghton Mifflin Company, 1957.

Smillie, W. *Public Health—Its Promise for the Future.* New York: The Macmillan Company, 1955.

Stewart, I. *The Education of Nurses.* New York: The Macmillan Company, 1950.

Strong, A. "The Education of Public Health Nurses." *The Public Health Nurse,* 13:226–30, May 1921.

Williams, R. C. *The United States Public Health Service.* Bethesda, Maryland: The Commissioned Officers Association of the United States Public Health Service, Box 5874, 1951.

Winslow C.-E. A. "Housing and Health." *The Public Health Nurse,* 32:434–39, July 1940.

CHAPTER 3

THE PERIOD FROM THE NEW DEAL THROUGH THE MID-1970S

The New Deal grew out of a shattering depression and brought with it a myriad of programs of relief, recovery, and reform designed to revitalize the machinery of a troubled nation. It resulted in a new role for the federal government—that of responsible overseer of the general welfare—and added a new dimension to social policy. It also resulted in more willingness on the part of the people to invest in common security at the expense of individual freedom.

The federal government demonstrated its real concern for the growing problems of the country. Between 1935 and the late sixties there was an increasing flow of legislation aimed at improvement of health and welfare, housing and urban development, antidiscrimination in civil rights, fair practices in employment, school desegregation, and aid to education, including nursing education. Ideas generated by the slogans "The New Frontier" of the Kennedy era and "The Great Society" of the subsequent Johnson era expressed the desire on the part of both the people and the government for an added dimension to the quality of life, and an expansion of opportunity and equality for all facets of society. Achievement of many of these ideas was not fully realized, in part because of the conservatism of the Nixon administration and the widening concern and disillusionment with America's deeper and deeper involvement in the undeclared and unpopular war in Vietnam. Elation over the end of the United States entanglement in the war was short lived, as the country was soon shocked by the Watergate affair and left with a pervasive disenchantment with its government. It felt a need to reassess values and goals. Blueprints for such plans as new towns, coordinated transportation systems, programs for the control of the environment, and restructured health and welfare systems were on the drawing boards.

Also, by the mid-1970s the country was well on its way to becoming an urban industrial society. Increases in population, transportation, and industrialization brought with them a whole new set of health and health-related problems. Some of these, such as environmental hazards, crime and delinquency, and drug addiction and its related problems, were a result of the shifting concentration of people. Nurses, along with other health professionals and consumers, were deeply involved in the problems and struggled to reevaluate and redefine their role and purposes to meet these new challenges. Nursing was firmly convinced that it must become truly professional, for only in this way could it integrate and utilize the results of rapid and expanding scientific, technologic, and sociologic knowledge, and with others meet the changing health needs of an impatient, better-educated, health-conscious people.

Nursing also increasingly valued higher education for nurses in contemporary society. By the mid-seventies it has set its sights in this direction and accepted baccalaureate education as beginning preparation for professional nursing, and graduate education as the base for the preparation of nurse specialists and leaders. Research and writing were gaining acceptance as important professional attributes. Nursing, along with other professions, was caught up in the universal struggle to make its education relevant.

Nurses, and particularly public health nurses, were participating with an expanding number of community health workers involved in planning and carrying out a complex of new and comprehensive health programs, both voluntary and governmental. As the pattern of health organization was changing, so was the role of nursing and public health nursing. The road ahead was exciting and challenging, but far from clear.

TRANSPORTATION

Transportation, which played so important a role on the early frontiers, was still a dominant factor in the increasing expansion of the country. By the beginning of World War II, the automobile had become a pivot for much of the life of the people. Production of automobiles came to a standstill during the war as many of the large automobile plants harnessed their machinery and workers to produce ships and airplanes.

After the war, however, production was resumed. In addition, advances in the design and construction of highways played a big part in the proliferation of the automobile. By the mid-seventies, the majority of American families owned at least one car, and many owned two. They were used for both business and pleasure.

The vast expansion of the automobile's domain had both good and bad effects, but there is no question about its impact on all aspects of life. The development of the cities, with the flight of the more affluent to the suburbs, could not have happened without the automobile. Parking problems, traffic congestion, violent deaths by accidents, noise, smog, and air pollution increased as the number of automobiles grew. The need for a huge network of more and better highways resulted in the bisection and dissection of farms and villages across the country by thousands of miles of superhighways. In spite of the number of highways, the production of cars outstripped road building, and traffic congestion magnified. As people moved to the suburbs, large shopping centers developed with ample parking facilities. At the same time, because of lack of parking facilities in some areas, many well-established stores in central cities either moved to suburban shopping centers or were forced to close their doors. Industry began to move out of the central cities as more and more people commuted to work by automobile and as industry became less dependent upon the railroads for transportation of goods and materials. The oil and gasoline crisis of 1974, precipitated by the decision of OPEC (the Organization of Petroleum Exporting Countries) to control the amount and cost of gasoline and oil available for import, shocked the country into recognition of its dependency on fuel importation and also its potential energy problem for the future. This resulted in

1. more government control of national fuel consumption and distribution
2. increased production and use of small cars
3. evaluation of real and potential national energy resources
4. energy conservation throughout the nation

It resulted, also, in reintroduction of the electric trolley, and increased research aimed at the development of alternative motor engines. There was renewed interest in the railroad as a more universal transportation system—a fact supported by federal legislation under the Federal Rail Reorganization Act. Concern over rising accident rates resulted in federal regulations regarding use of seat belts and provision of other safety measures in auto construction.

Mobility continued to be a way of life. Gone were the days when a child was born, lived out his lifespan, and died in the same community.

Goods and produce were accessible to everyone, even in some of the remotest parts of the country. At the same time television, radio, and other mass media were constantly reminding the people of the things they could have or that others had. New industries and occupations developed to keep the transportation system operating and to meet the needs of the people for recreational activities made possible by developments in transportation.

The airplane was still in its infancy at the outbreak of World War II hostilities, but the needs of the war hastened its development. Within less than three decades after the war, commercial airlines expanded, jet planes which could transport large numbers of people around the world in a matter of hours became commonplace, and travel to the moon was a reality. Airports were developed in or adjacent to all the major cities. By the mid-seventies air congestion had become a serious problem, and the need for more and larger airports to accommodate the superjets and their increased number of passengers was a source of concern. With the increased speed of transportation more stringent methods of disease surveillance became necessary because of the rapidity with which disease could spread from one part of the world to another. The noise-abatement program to reduce the sound of airplanes became a major occupation. Controversy over noise and pollution from supersonic planes was intense—resulting in only grudging permission to allow the French supersonic *Concorde* to land in one American airport.

In the expansion of transportation there was a partnership between the federal government and private enterprise, with each dependent upon the other. The federal government subsidized highway construction over which the automobile, developed by private enterprise, traveled. Government weather forecasts and air-traffic control were necessary in order for commercial airlines to operate. National and international regulations to control the spread of disease made it possible for airplanes to carry people to all corners of the world. Federal subsidy of railroads made it possible for the railroads to survive during the period of declining traffic. Government expenditures and controls made possible the voluntary coordination of the industrialists to develop the means to meet the needs of the people for transportation.

INDUSTRIALIZATION AND TECHNOLOGY

During the depression years industrial expansion had been practically nil, and many industries cut back production to a minimum. Unemployment soared, and the plight of the workers was desperate. Labor unions, which had been struggling unsuccessfully to organize workers on a nationwide basis, were able to flourish in this climate.

Legislation favorable to the development of strong labor unions was enacted, and the organization of workers in their own behalf was sanctioned by the nation for the first time.

By the beginning of the Second World War, production of goods had resumed, industry was on its way to recovery, and crippling strikes by labor unions were a threat to be reckoned with. Production of domestic goods came to a halt at the outbreak of the war, with the entire industrial and technologic power geared to the war effort. A moratorium on strikes was declared by the labor unions and was one of the factors which contributed to the enormous industrial and technologic growth during the war years. The government and universities collaborated in joint ventures for the development of scientific research and technology to meet the tremendous needs of modern warfare. Once again the American genius for know-how and the practical ingenuity of the people came to the fore. Automobile factories became airplane factories, ships were built at a phenomenal rate, increases in agriculture revolutionized farming, synthetic rubber was developed, new drugs such as penicillin appeared almost daily, strides were made in the treatment of the sick and wounded, and radar was developed and used extensively. The race for atomic weapons was won by the United States, and the war came to an end when atom bombs were dropped on Hiroshima and Nagasaki. The atom bomb ushered in the nuclear age, and a worldwide contest began for supremacy in the development of greater and more devastating war weapons. This contest was destined to change the power structure of the world.

After the war the economy shifted to the production of consumer goods. People who had "done without" for so many years clamored for all sorts of products. The supply at first was small, and inflation was an ever-present threat. The no-strike policy of the labor unions ended, and devastating strikes crippled most of the major industries. In 1947 Congress passed the Taft-Hartley Act in an effort to dilute some of the power of organized labor. There was much opposition to this legislation by the labor unions, and the controversy is still going on today.

The development and expansion of television after the war was probably more important to the country than the expansion of the radio had been after World War I. Dulles[1] estimates that in 1958 there were 50,000,000 television sets in use. Television was bringing into the living room every type of entertainment and spectator sport, political contests, educational programs, war, and commercials. No facet of life was immune. For the first time people were seeing what they were missing, and their desires and aspirations were changed. The distance between the rich and the poor became more visible. At the same time the American people enjoyed a higher standard of living than the world had ever known. Mass distribution of goods was as important as mass production. People in all walks of life were buying and using the same commodities, seeing the same kinds of shows, reading the same kinds of books, riding in the same kinds of automobiles, and traveling to the same places. There were differences in the degree to which people participated, but no longer was participation only for an elite group.

Scientific and technologic discoveries, which in peacetime might have taken many years, advanced at a phenomenal rate during World War II and helped to trigger a whole new concern over environmental health. Development of nerve gas, development and use of DDT and other pesticides, and important biologic research such as that in oceanography had unexpected and frightening results. For example, in the fifties scientists began to uncover disturbing facts about DDT's effects on the chain of life—its tendency to accumulate in the fatty tissue of wildlife. Questions were raised about the effect of pesticides even deadlier than DDT in regard to sporadically reported fish kills. The relationship of all of this to human life was disturbingly unclear.

Also in the fifties, Sweden reported high death rates among birds which had eaten methylmercury-coated seeds. Mysteriously fatal "epidemics" among humans were tracked down to methylmercury-coated seeds in Iraq in 1956, in West Pakistan in 1961, and in Guatemela in 1963.[2]

Rachael Carson's book *Silent Spring* was published in 1962. As a literary work having impact upon a great social debate, it has been likened to Harriet Beecher Stowe's *Uncle Tom's Cabin.* Robert Rudd, a noted biologist, said of the book:

> *Silent Spring* is biological warning, social commentary and moral reminder. Insistently she calls upon technological man to pause and take stock.[3]

By 1962 people were growing increasingly apprehensive over reports about environment hazards. *Silent Spring* gave focus and meaning to a swelling debate and discussion of the issues. The issues involved even more than the immediate and long-range effects of pesticides and methylmercury. They included, and still include, not only the whole problem of the pollution of the air, water, and food, but also the ultimate destruction of the very planet. They involve reevaluation of the quality of life itself. Nelson A. Rockefeller, governor of New York and later vice-president of the United States, said:

> By 1970 we have explored almost every square mile of this planet. We have begun to explore the lunar satellite and the more remote

> areas of the sea bed. We are planning a "grand tour" of the other planets, much in the mode of a photographic safari. We have explored the microcosm to the smallest subparticle of matter, split the atom, probed the secrets of chromosomes and genes and, through them, the key to life itself. "But with all our relentless searching for knowledge," as Ewald B. Nyquist, New York State Commissioner of Education, has put it, "we have forgotten that man himself is the ultimate reason for our eternal quest, and that the individual is still the basic unit of value in the human condition."[4]

By the mid-seventies, the enormous expansion of science and technology had changed the whole structure of society. The economy had shifted from the production of goods to the provision of services, such as health, recreation, and education. The nuclear age had been replaced by the space age. Man had walked on the moon. Interstellar probes had been launched into space and a satellite had landed on Mars. Both men and women were applying for positions on the first space shuttle. It was still generally accepted that science and technology could solve many problems of the times. The very secrets of life were being explored, with the discovery of DNA and RNA opening up undreamed vistas. By the mid-seventies, however, legislation was being proposed to limit or even halt genetic research, for fear of dire consequences.

Several new kinds of relationships evolved as a result of the development of a technology-industry-research triad. As the country assumed a more military stance during the fifties and became involved first in the Korean War and subsequently in the struggle in Vietnam and Southeast Asia, a whole new industrial-military complex came into being. There was a marked interest in government contracts with industry for production of military supplies and equipment, and with both industry and educational institutions for research relative to the war effort. Industry, particularly the military-industrial complex which had been enhanced by our involvement in the Vietnam War, was a powerful influence on the economic stability of the country. The conversion of industry after Vietnam from meeting the needs of the military to meeting the needs of the people contributed to a rising unemployment rate. A substantial number of unemployed were those with research knowledge and talents who had developed the complex technology that was responsible for their unemployment. Powerful labor unions, with their ever-increasing demands, were playing havoc with the economy and contributing to inflation and unemployment.

A new partnership between technology and medicine grew by leaps and bounds. Developments in medical technology of such aids as heart pacemakers, hydrodialysis equipment, artificial organs, and hyperbaric chambers revolutionized medical and surgical care. Of no less importance to medical science were the results of genetic research and the development of myriad new drugs.

Other technologic advances which evolved, such as the computer, were beginning to create in people the feeling that society was becoming depersonalized. Fear was being expressed about the future influence of technology and scientific advances on the very fabric of life. The compatibility of technology with the quality of life was unclear, and many feared that technology might get first priority. Some of this concern was caused by the impossibility of keeping up with the expansion of knowledge. In 1964, Bell estimated that 50,000 technical journals with 1,200,000 articles were published annually, and that major libraries would double their holdings every 16 years.[5] In all of this knowledge revolution a higher premium was being placed on education: if one does not understand what is going on he cannot participate: this in turn adds to the depersonalization.

POPULATION

The impact of World War II on migration was pronounced, and mobility in general was characteristic and widespread. Job opportunities in defense establishments mushroomed, and unemployment practically disappeared. There was a mass movement of black families from the South to the North seeking employment. Thousands of individuals and families were uprooted—moving from the country to the city for defense jobs, participation in the whole war effort, or both in combination. Many of these never returned to their original homes, and the urban situation never returned to its prewar state.

Immigration after 1930 no longer made any significant contribution to the population increase. However, after the war Puerto Ricans in growing numbers came to the States and, more specifically, to New York City. The Puerto Rican was handicapped in the American city—more so than the earlier immigrants. His previous life was rural; he could not speak English, was unskilled, and had few financial resources. As a group, Puerto Ricans did not have the cohesiveness and optimistic outlook that was a characteristic of the earlier immigrants.

The plight of the cities continued to worsen in the seventies, with the constant immigration of blacks and Puerto Ricans into the center city, and the emigration of the more affluent to the suburbs. The ghetto areas of the cities bore some resemblance to the slum areas of earlier periods. Poverty, poor housing, lack of recreational facilities, illiteracy resulting from language barriers, poor transportation facilities, and poor health made excellent breeding grounds for crime and delinquency. Drugs and drug pushers flourished. High infant death rates in some census tracts were indicative of the lack of availability or utilization of health care by the people. In contrast to the earlier periods, the aspirations of the people had been heightened by federal legislation, such as the War on Poverty and the legal definition of poverty. Television, also, had increased the thirst of the people for their share of available goods. They were more oriented to the present than their parents and grandparents (who were willing to tolerate bad conditions because of the promise of a better life in the future), and were demanding immediate solutions to their problems. Skin color made upward mobility difficult and increased the smoldering resentment of the ghetto dwellers. The ingredients for a conflagration were present and waiting to be touched off unless drastic intervention on a large scale was undertaken. In some cities, tensions and violence flared as a result of forced busing being used as a tool for racial integration of schools. Traffic congestion, poor public transportation, rising tax rates, high rents, and bureaucratic forms of city government contributed to the movement of industry and people to the suburbs. Increasingly, cities were becoming overwhelmed by the poor, the elderly, and the transients, with costs for welfare and other forms of relief rising steadily with no end in sight. The flow of the middle class to the suburbs, and from the suburbs to the semisuburbs, accelerated. Some of the reasons for this were a steadily rising income level, a better standard of living, more automobiles, and improved roads. The availability of single housing units, better schools, and more widespread middle-class manners and morals gave people a feeling that the suburbs were a better place in which to raise a family. As a group, suburbanites constituted the largest number of people in the nation. The implications of this group as a political and legislative bloc were beginning to be more fully understood.

The movement to the suburbs further increased the plight of the cities. American cities have always been plagued with the problems of the underprivileged, and the situation continues to worsen. Increased migration with security of adequate low- and middle-income housing, inadequate transportation, poor parking facilities, traffic congestion, overcrowding, noise, and smog make the city a less desirable place in which to live. Between 1950 and 1960, more than three-quarters of the metropolitan growth took place outside the central city—and the poor rushed in to fill the void. Poverty, not exclusively a result of urbanization, remained primarily a problem of the central cities and certain rural districts of the country. The conditions of the poor, although not as desperate as those of the earlier immigrants in the slums, were in sharp contrast to those of an increasing number of Americans who by the end of the sixties enjoyed the most affluent society the world has ever known.

By the mid-1970s, the population had reached 204 million. The rate of population growth, 18 percent between 1950 and 1960, began to decelerate and between 1960 and 1970 grew by 13 percent. Bureau of the Census estimates for 1980 show an increase over 1970 that may drop to 8 percent.[8] The need for population control was uppermost in the minds of many. Controversy over which were the best methods to accomplish this was worldwide. In the United States, pros and cons of various approaches were aired in the press. The constitutionality of some of the state laws limiting or prohibiting birth control was being challenged in the Supreme Court. Federal money was available to enable state and local communities to establish family-planning programs. Abortion laws were becoming less restrictive. The birth rate had declined from 25.2 per thousand in 1957 to 14.9 per thousand in 1973.[7] Between 1960 and 1972 life expectancy at birth had increased from 66.7 to 67.4 years for men and from 73.1 to 75.2 years for women.[8]

EDUCATION

During the depression public school attendance burgeoned. Lunch programs were introduced into some of the public schools in an effort to alleviate hunger and to prevent some of the ravages of malnutrition. In 1935, the National Youth Administration (NYA) was established to provide training for unemployed youth and part-time employment for needy students. As unemployment increased and fewer jobs were available for young people, more and more of them attended high school.

By 1947, practically all the children between 6 and 13 years of age were in elementary school; 81.2 percent of the 14-to-17-year age group were in high school; and half of the 25-to-29-year age group had 12 or more years of schooling.[9].

In 1954, the Supreme Court ruled against separate but equal education for blacks and directed the states to desegregate their schools "with all deliberate speed." There was much resistance to this decision, and the legislators in several of the southern states enacted laws in an attempt to circumvent it. The exact meaning of the phrase "with all deliberate speed" was unclear and was interpreted differently by each individual and group. Token integration occurred, but the majority of black children were educated in segregated schools.

By 1970, elementary and secondary education had become a necessity for everyone, and a high school education was a prerequisite for even the unskilled worker. Boys and girls were educated together, both in the cities and the rural areas. However, in contrast to the earlier period when the quality of public school education in the cities was superior to that of other areas, a reverse situation was occurring. The movement of middle-class people from the cities to the suburbs and the migration of blacks, Puerto Ricans, and unskilled workers to the cities confronted the schools with an almost impossible task. It was difficult to recruit well-prepared teachers to the ghetto schools, the children in the schools came from families that were socially and culturally deprived, and the curricula were not relevant to the concerns of the increasing number of people in the lower socioeconomic group.

As the number of high school students grew, there was a proportionate demand for college education. This demand had an impact on the expansion of the junior college movement. Junior colleges, or community colleges, as they were sometimes called, made it possible for more students to live at home and to pursue further education. For the most part the curriculum consisted of the first two years of a baccalaureate program. In the fifties, the junior colleges turned their attention to meeting the needs of the people in their own community. Vocational curricula and adult education were added to the offerings. By 1959 there were 390 public and 273 private junior colleges with a total enrollment of 816,071.[10]

By 1939, the estimated college enrollment was 1,365,000,[11] and the attitude of the public toward higher education had changed. The National Youth Administration with its student work administration program made it possible for needy students to defray some of the costs of higher education. This was the first substantial federal program to assist students to attend college. There was a growing awareness that the nation's people were its prime resource, and that national security and welfare were dependent upon a high level of education and skill.

The war, with all its myriad demands, mobilized the nation and further emphasized the need for highly educated people. Because of the needs of science and technology, a new relationship developed between higher education and the federal government. The Serviceman's Readjustment Act, familiarly known as the G.I. Bill, which was passed in 1944, is often referred to as the Morrill Act of the twentieth century. To date no other single program has had so great an impact on American higher education. College enrollment swelled, and in 1947, the peak year of veteran enrollment, one and one-half million, or roughly one-half of all college students were veterans. For the most part, the veterans were serious students who were more concerned with obtaining an education than with extracurricular activities. Many were married, and their wives and children lived with them on college campuses throughout the country. There was much concern that total college enrollment would drop after the peak years of the veterans. This did not occur, however, as by then the value of higher education for all who could benefit from it had become a pervading value of American society.

By the early sixties, college enrollment had reached 4,880,000, and 35 percent of the people between 18 and 21 years of age were in college.[12] The majority of the students by this time were enrolled in coeducational public institutions, with the largest numbers still from the upper socioeconomic groups. However, scholarships from colleges and universities, from philanthropic foundations, from industry, and from the state and federal governments were becoming more readily available, thus making it possible for more young people from lower socioeconomic groups to attend college. By this time, the focus of higher education had shifted from one of personal development to one of social responsibility. The relevancy of the curriculum to meet this responsibility was being challenged, and students were beginning to demand more freedom in planning their own course of study.

Graduate and professional education expanded, spurred by the passage of the National Defense Education Act of 1958, which provided federal support to students in graduate and undergraduate school. This was the first tangible step by the federal government to ensure that each individual have the opportunity to receive the most advanced education for which he qualified in order to assure the well-being of the nation. Graduate education was becoming a prerequisite for many top-level positions in management, teaching, and administration.

The federal government was turning more and more to the universities to promote specific goals of the country, such as research, training of personnel, and consultation. Scientists and scholars were being drawn more and more into world affairs. However, there was no overall federal policy or goal for higher education as a whole, as was true in some of the other countries of the world.

By the late sixties, student unrest and turmoil were characteristic phenomena of the times, and universities were one of their prime targets. The degree of student discontent seemed to parallel the increasing involvement of the country in the Vietnam War, and criticism focused on military-related university involvement, such as ROTC programs and government-sponsored university research relative to the war effort. In addition, student unrest and involvement with the whole civil rights movement resulted in efforts to increase the number of black university students and faculty as well as develop black studies programs. A general and growing discontent on the part of university students with the country in general, and the irrelevancy of their university education in particular, resulted in widespread student demonstrations, strikes, and frightening violence. Students demanded and assumed much more involvement with both curriculum planning and a widening range of decisions relative to higher education.

After the United States involvement in the Vietnam War came to an end, the militancy of students in institutions of higher education lessened—almost to the point of apathy. The focus of student concern shifted to relevance of education, preparation for employment, rising costs, and availability of more nontraditional learning opportunities. The number of part-time students, and those in work-study and atypical programs, increased.

The cost of education on all levels rose dramatically, and in many states it was the largest item in the budget, accounting for one-quarter of the financial expenditure of state monies. However, there was much discussion and debate about the role of the federal government in financing and in improving the quality of education.

The first comprehensive federal legislation to provide funds for nursing education was the Nurse Training Act of 1964, which added Title VIII, Nurse Training, to the Public Health Service Act. Title VIII was designed to improve nursing education, with the objective of encouraging the education of nurses in appropriate numbers capable of providing quality nursing care whenever it was needed. Title VIII authorized grants for construction of nursing education facilities, projects to improve nurse training, formula payments for diploma schools, and low-cost, partially cancelable loans for nursing students. The Professional Nurse Traineeship program, established in 1956, was continued under this Title, and broadened to include advanced education in clinical specialities.

The Health Manpower Act of 1968, Title II, broadened the nurse training provisions and extended the authority for two years—fiscal years 1970 through 1971. The Nurse Training Act of 1971 expanded and extended federal aid to nursing education through June 1974. These additions were included: basic support in the form of capitation grants to schools of nursing that expand their enrollments and provide education to prepare certain types of nurse practitioners; separate authorities for financial-distress grants to schools of nursing; and start-up grants for new nurse training programs.[13]

The federal government, thus, had been assisting nursing in a variety of ways to improve the supply, quality, education, and distribution of nurses—and thus improve health care for the nation. By the mid-seventies, however, there was less federal support for higher education—due, perhaps, in part to the backlash from earlier campus unrest.

The financial plight of private colleges and universities was acute, and rising tuition threatened to restrict private education to the affluent. A large majority of college students were in coeducational institutions. In the sixties, many men's and women's colleges, as well as private proprietary schools, had become coeducational in their own right or through affiliation with another institution. By the mid-seventies, however, this trend was changing, and both men's and women's colleges were less willing to open their doors to both sexes. The number of women attending college increased after the decline in the late fifties and sixties. By the seventies, it was generally accepted that women had equal rights to higher education, but they still did not have equal access in relation to such areas as admissions, courses of study, and job opportunities. The question and problem of providing equal educational opportunity without regard to sex, age, race, or any other class identification persisted. Federal affirmative action legislation was resulting in some slow progress.

WOMEN

Participation of women in the labor force prior to World War II increased significantly, but the war itself changed the entire picture. Unemployment was reduced practically overnight, and large numbers of women went to work. As in the Civil War and World War I, they took many jobs that had previously been open only to men. Many were recruited and trained for complicated technical production-line and service responsibilities. Others, who previously had been involved full time with their homes and families, devoted their energies to myriad voluntary services needed for the war effort. Women for the first time joined all branches of the armed forces and had the same military rank and pay as men. By the end of the war there were 16,000,000 women in the labor force.[14] This pattern of women working full time did not change, and the proportion of married women working outside the home increased each year. Mowry states[15] that by 1960 more than one-third of women of working age were either employed or looking for work. Within some age groups, 28 percent of the married women were working.

The struggle by women for equality in American society, characterized by such purpose and vitality earlier in the century, was gaining momentum slowly. Very little progress had been made by midcentury. In fact, women seemed to have lost ground in their battle for equality of opportunity. This occurred in spite of the fact that changes in the pattern of marriage, child rearing, and life span had resulted in more time available to women for full-time employment or career development outside the home.

By 1957, the median age at which a girl left school was 18, she married at 20, and had her last child at 26. She was 32 by the time her youngest child went to school, and her life expectancy was 79 years of age.[16] There was general acceptance that women had the same right as men to higher education. They had proved they had the mental capacity and the physical endurance. There was not, however, general acceptance that higher education was equally important for women as for men, and women had not continued to take equal advantage of this opportunity. Some of the women were also questioning the value of their college education, and the early pioneering for women's education had lost most of its momentum. During the fifties and early sixties there was a slow but steady decline in the proportion of women enrolled in programs of higher education. By the mid-seventies research still indicates that women continued to be underrepresented in the college-going population, with the national ratio per hundred entering freshmen now standing at 54 men to 45 women.[17]

Of particular interest were the changes in the pattern of involvement of women in the economy of the country, in higher education, and in the mainstream of American society in general. The fact of greater participation of women in the labor force was unquestionable. However, in many instances upward job opportunity was not available, and there were often salary inequities for men and women in the same jobs. In spite of an increasing number of career women, very few of these were in administrative, legislative, or policy-making positions. These roles still remained male bastions. Promotions for women were fewer than for men, and they did not receive equal pay for equal work.

The majority of professional women were nurses or teachers, and most of this latter group were found in the elementary schools. Few were high-school principals. Those who were employed by colleges and universities taught predominantly within professional schools of nursing, education, or social work, or were in women's colleges. The numbers with top university administrative responsibilities continued to be so small as to be almost insignificant. A look at responsible positions in government, politics, and professions such as law, medicine, and engineering revealed the same lack of participation by women.

By 1960, it was evident that women had not tried to consolidate and extend their claim to equality from the vote to fuller participation in the affairs of the country. They appeared to have a lack of commitment to full-time meaningful employment. The conflict between the goal of home and family versus career continued, and was enhanced by the still-prevalent view of society that "woman's place is in the home." On the other hand, society was beginning to change its attitude toward women's goals and to recognize their great potential contribution to a society which needed the best of all its citizens. Civil rights legislation passed by Congress included the elimination of discrimination in the employment of women. More and more of the material wealth of the country was controlled by women, and their full participation in the economy was increasingly important. By the mid-seventies, however, there had been a resurgence of the women's rights movement. The Equal Rights Amendment was being considered for ratification by the various state legislatures. The women's rights movement was intensifying and was demonstrating a militancy akin to that of the Civil Rights movement. Progress was hard to measure, but one had a feeling of small gains and gradual change.

SOCIAL CONSCIOUSNESS

Historians say that the depression years were the most disastrous period in the history of the country. There was widespread despair, cynicism, questioning, hunger, and suffering. On the other hand, the depression and the years following had a profound effect on the already ingrained social consciousness of the American people. They were deeply affected by the plight of so many of their fellow countrymen and readily accepted and supported programs provided for the poor, the unemployed, and the helpless victims of circumstances well beyond their control. More people than ever before participated in a variety of voluntary efforts and helped to raise large sums of money for relief and welfare. Paralleling these voluntary efforts was the ever-growing involvement of the federal government in programs for the general welfare, with the role of the voluntary organization a complementary one. There seemed to be a change in society as a whole, resulting in a willingness on the part of the people to invest in the common good, even at the expense of the individual. This shift in emphasis was reflected also in the general attitude toward education. Where formerly education had been considered of value primarily for growth of the individual, its importance for the social development of the country was now recognized.

The post-World War II years were less turbulent than those following World War I. Perhaps one of the reasons for this was that the people were more realistic about the results of war and not as emotionally entangled with slogans such as "a war to end all wars" or "a war to make the world safe for democracy." They clamored and worked for the good things in life, but the social consciousness that had been reawakened during the depression and had changed the whole fabric of American life could not be ignored. The role of the federal government in the life of the people increased, with each Congress outdoing the other in the amount of social legislation it enacted. The distance between the "haves" and "have-nots" became more visible with the nationwide spread of television, and there was a pervasive feeling that the good things in life should be available to all. There was no general consensus, however, about how this should be accomplished. Some felt that the government should assume more responsibility; while others feared too much federal involvement.

National voluntary organizations grew by leaps and bounds, and the generosity of the American people in contributing to innumerable and sundry appeals for funds became legendary. The community chest, which had developed after the First World War, became firmly established in almost every community, and the red feather, which was its symbol, became a familiar sight.

"The New Frontier," the slogan of the Kennedy administration in the early sixties, set the stage for progress in social welfare, housing, civil rights, and education. The ringing words of the president, "ask not what your country can do for you, ask what you can do for your country," expressed the mood of the early sixties—one of idealism, hope, and commitment.

The Peace Corps gave hundreds of Americans the opportunity to become personally involved in helping the less fortunate in other parts of the world. Volunteers in Service to America (VISTA) provided the means through which people could serve those within the country itself—the less fortunate, the poor, and the elderly.

During the Kennedy era there was a desire for change and a feeling, particularly on the part of youth, that change was possible. The country was able to take a giant step forward, the greatest since the Civil War, toward equality for blacks with its civil rights legislation. In areas where federal power could be evoked, government support was received, Sit-ins, demonstrations, and attacks on de facto segregation and discrimination in schools, public transportation, housing, and employment swept across the country. The courage and inspiration of Martin Luther King, Jr., immortalized by both his Nobel Peace Prize and his assassination, touched the hearts of Americans. Larry L. King wrote of the Kennedy influence in April 1968:

> We needed something. Kennedy gave it to us. Call it a sense of style. Suddenly America might be believed again. It might grow young. Its liver spots might disappear. It might reach the moon and other high destinies; young men and women of many races and classes joined hands in the bloodier thickets of the South and sang their hope. We Shall Overcome. Our youth invaded distant lands not with flame-throwers and guns but as missionaries of the Peace Corps. Appalachia would come to life; Martin Luther King would have his dream; America was on the move again. How incredibly naive it all seems today, and how quickly it passed.[18]

The youth of the country were very much involved in the civil rights movement. Their concern soon spread to other issues, such as war and peace, poverty, and basic values of the individual and society.

"The Great Society" slogan of the Johnson era signified the path which the country chose to continue to follow after the Kennedy assassination—and extended and expanded federal legislation and support for the elimination of poverty and inequality. By 1964, some of the barriers against discrimination were beginning to crumble, but racial tensions were exploding as the contrast between affluence and poverty came into sharper and sharper focus. Legislation establishing the Office of Economic Opportunity and the resultant poverty programs supported the development of hundreds of community health- and welfare-oriented programs aimed at improving services, particularly for those in densely populated cities across the nation. Involvement of citizens in planning and carrying out these services was an important aspect of the poverty program.

Increasing dissatisfaction with the Vietnam war paralleled deepening involvement in the southeast Asian conflict—and the mood of the country began to change from one of hope to one of pessimism. The inspiration of the Kennedy era no longer existed, and an inspiration gap developed during the Johnson era.

Student unrest was growing, and in the late sixties its focus shifted from the national scene to the campus. Campus involvement in ROTC and military research were major concerns at first. Soon, wave after wave of student violence swept across the campuses—aimed at war, inequality, the Establishment, middle-class values, and alleged irrelevance of education. By the end of the sixties, changes within the educational system had occurred and students were much involved in decision-making on important issues. There were many people across the country who disagreed with student goals, methods, and aims. Lee, in discussing the college student, says,

> Each generation discovers its own gods, its own high priests, its own answers. Each generation grapples in its own way with the problems of war, injustice, sex, and job security and through its struggles with these, each generation defines its own ethos.[19]

The Nixon era will no doubt be recorded as a dark time in the history of America. It was a time of retrenchment and drying up of federal funds for the support of a variety of health and welfare programs. Continued involvement in the increasingly unpopular Vietnam War had resulted in preoccupation with foreign affairs rather than concern for domestic problems. Elation at the long hoped-for disentanglement of the United States from the war had faded rapidly with the Watergate scandal and the subsequent resignation of the president. The country, visibly shaken by the events, experienced a sense of shock that Watergate could have happened at the very heart of its government. There was a pervasive feeling of disenchantment with the government. There was also a feeling of pride in the fact that the country had survived such a crisis. By the mid-seventies a deeply concerned, socially conscious America was again struggling to redefine its values and goals. This was not easy within a time of accelerating change. The issues of major concern were not so different from those with which other generations had grappled in earlier periods, but the solutions—to remain viable—would have to endure within the changing world of the eighties and the future.

NURSING

Nurses did not escape the impact of the depression, and many were forced to join the growing ranks of the unemployed. Their need for full-time, or even part-time work, was desperate. It did, however, aid in the solution of one of the problems which had plagued nursing for a long time—the fact that the bulk of nursing care to patients in hospitals was given by students, with the result that the quality of care left much to be desired. As employment of graduate nurses in hospitals increased, so did their concern about the need to improve the care their patients were receiving. Poor working conditions and long hours of work added to their dissatisfaction. Wages and working conditions of other workers were receiving top billing by some of the labor unions, and many groups were demanding equitable salaries. The American Nurses' Association, in 1946, launched an economic security program for nurses that was aimed at remedying some of the inequities in the employment of nurses. There was much furor about whether this was a function of a professional organization. It was not until the early sixties that the problems of employed nurses were brought to the attention of the nation. By this time other professional organizations, such as the National Education Association, were also demanding changes in the remuneration and working conditions of their members. What began as a palliative measure to provide employment for nurses during the depression resulted in real concern about and recognition of the need to provide better care to patients and better working conditions for nurses. Staffing patterns changed, and the 8-hour day became a reality for many nurses. By the end of World War II the graduate nurse was recognized as an accepted member of the hospital staff, and it was difficult to imagine a hospital without her.

Growing concern over the quality of nursing care contributed to reevaluation of the educational programs which were preparing these nurses. The Curriculum Guide of 1937 had recommended that psychiatric nursing be included in the education of all nurses, and also pointed the way for needed reform in nursing education. Changes and improvements were occurring: high school graduation became a requirement for admission to schools of nursing; many poor diploma schools closed; and the number of programs within institutions of higher education showed an increase. The long-to-be-continued controversy over the kind and amount of clinical practice necessary for student learning began at this time.

When World War II started, nursing had already taken steps to meet the demands of the military and the civilian population. The American Nurses' Association, the National League for Nursing Education, and the National Organization for Public Health Nursing, early in 1940, held a joint convention in Philadelphia to discuss steps to be taken. Following this meeting, the Nursing Council of National Defense was formed with representatives from the Army and Navy Nurse Corps, the Children's Bureau, the Veterans Administration, the Indian Service, the United States Public Health Service, the national nursing organizations, and the American Red Cross. This council became the National Nursing Council for War Service after war was declared. Some of its concerns were to increase and assure the supply of nursing students; to help in the equitable distribution of graduate nurses for both the armed forces and the home front; and to make greater use of auxiliary nurses. It was also concerned about such things as working hours, wages, and living conditions for nurses.

During the war many nurses joined the Army and Navy Nurse Corps. At the same time women in large numbers were joining other branches of the armed forces. To assure a continuous supply of nurses, federal legislation was passed establishing the Cadet Nurse Corps. Students enrolled in the Cadet Corps had their tuition and fees paid and received a monthly living allowance. In addition, hospital uniforms were supplied as well as an outdoor uniform. Many young women were attracted to the Cadet Nurse Corps, and by the end of the war the total enrollment reached 179,000, with approximately 95 percent of all nursing students members of the Corps.[20] Funds were included in the bill establishing the Cadet Corps, for the preparation of teaching and supervisory personnel to meet the expanded enrollment. The administration of the funds was the responsibility of a Division of Nurse Education in the United States Public Health Service. In 1944, a Division of Nursing was established in the Public Health Service and given jurisdiction and general supervision for all nursing in the Public Health Service—another milestone in the development of nursing in the United States.

After the war, the demand for health services and health personnel was insatiable, as patients poured into hospitals, clinics, and medical centers. Although no overall national health plan had been developed, prepayment plans for hospital care were growing by leaps and bounds. The impact on nursing of new and rapidly expanding scientific knowledge, and developments in medical technique, resulted in the assumption by the nurse of an increasing number of tasks formerly considered to be the responsibility of the physician.

Application of continuing advances in medical science and technology demanded a high degree of nursing as well as medical skill and knowledge. Patterns of delivery of patient care were changing, and utilization of health resources increased markedly. People were better informed regarding health and accepted it as a right.

Many nurses who had been in the armed forces took advantage of the educational opportunity provided by the G.I. Bill and enrolled full time in colleges and universities. The number of nurses with a college education was greater than it had ever been. The kinds and numbers of nurses needed to meet the changing needs of society, and how these nurses were to be educated, were of constant concern to nursing. The National Nursing Council, as one of its last activities before disbanding in 1948, was responsible for the launching of the now-famous study known as the Brown Report.[21]

Brown reported that persons conversant with the trends in professional education in the United States were practically unanimous in the opinion that the preparation of professional nurses belonged in institutions of higher learning. She advocated that the nonprofessional nurse be accepted and prepared within public vocational schools, that poor diploma schools close, and that the good ones make every effort to further improve their curricula. They should also experiment in simultaneously shortening the period of education while improving the course of study. Especially recommended as transitional steps toward the future were the creation of central schools of nursing and the utilization of the teaching resources of junior colleges. The Brown Report recommended:

> that nursing make one of its first matters of important business the long overdue official examination of every school; that the list of accredited schools be published and distributed as far as possible to every town and city of the United States.[22]

This report gave added impetus and a sense of direction to midcentury nursing educational reform. The pervading feeling in society of the need for educated people to meet society's needs was penetrating nursing, and nursing education was moving into institutions of higher learning. Since the beginning of the war, the American Association of Junior Colleges and the National Council for War Services had been thinking together about collaborating further in the education of nurses, as many prenursing courses were available in junior colleges.

In 1951, Mildred Montag's[23] dissertation was used as a model for the development of community college education for nurses. The relationship between community colleges and nursing, at first experimental, became well established as a viable pattern of nursing education. Many of the fears and concerns expressed when the experiment started began to be alleviated.

The structure of the six nursing organizations was cumbersome, and problems of coordination were increasing. After considerable study of the structure of the existing organizations, a plan of merger and reorganization was accepted in 1952. The merger resulted in two companion organizations. One was the American Nurses' Association, whose main purposes were the continuing improvement of professional practice and the economic and general welfare of nurses. Membership was open only to registered nurses. The other organization was the National League for Nursing, whose purposes were for nurses and friends of nursing to work together, to provide the best possible nursing services to people, and to assure good nursing education. Membership was open to nurses and lay persons alike. A Coordinating Council was established to coordinate programs of common concern to the American Nurses' Association and the National League for Nursing, and to keep in touch with each other's work. At the same time, the National Student Nurse Association was organized under the guidance of both the American Nurses' Association and the National League for Nursing.

The quality of nursing education programs and how to evaluate them had long been of concern to the National League for Nursing Education. In 1937, a committee on accreditation had been established in which the National League for Nursing Education, the Association of Collegiate Schools of Nursing, and the National Organization for Public Health Nursing worked closely together to evaluate programs in nursing education. In spite of close collaboration, there was much overlapping of activity within these three groups. Finally, in 1948, the National Nursing Accreditation Service was organized. It was responsible for the accreditation of all nursing programs. Four boards of review were established—one for basic noncollegiate professional nursing education, one for basic collegiate nursing education, one for public health nursing, and one for postgraduate professional nursing education. In 1953, the responsibility for the accreditation of nursing programs was transferred to the newly formed National League for Nursing. Criteria for accreditation, and the whole process and procedure have been constantly evaluated and revised over the years in line with changes and developments in nursing and nursing education. For example, in 1958, the following decisions were made:

1. That the National League for Nursing no longer accredit educational programs which provide specialization at the baccalaureate level.
2. That the National League for Nursing accredit only those baccalaureate programs which include psychiatric nursing.
3. That after five years the National League for Nursing accredit only those baccalaureate programs which include public health nursing.
4. That the National League for Nursing seek assistance of the National Commission on Accrediting to halt development of unsound programs.[24]

Nursing took leadership in its program of accreditation which has been a model for other accreditation groups. It established collaborative relationships with six of the regional associations in higher education—North Central, Middle Atlantic States, Southern, New England, Northwest, and Western. For many years the National Commission on Accrediting has recognized the National League for Nursing as responsible for voluntary accreditation of baccalaureate and higher degree programs in nursing.

Licensure for the practice of nursing was one concern of the American Nurses' Association. The state of New York which, in 1938, had enacted a law requiring licensing of all who nurse for hire, was a pioneer in this endeavor. The law established two groups—one for registered nurses and the other for licensed practical nurses. This law, suspended during the war, was reenacted in 1949, at which time its mandatory provisions came into full effect. The question of a national licensing system, discussed many times, has run into states' rights as a stumbling block. All states have licensing laws, most of which are mandatory, but there are still a few which are permissive. Each state developed its own state board examination questions until 1944. At that time the National League for Nursing Education developed examinations which could be used by all the states. These examinations, known as the State Board Test Pool, are controlled by the Council of State Boards, which is under the jurisdiction of the American Nurses' Association.

Of deep concern to nurses during the seventies was the whole question of individual versus institutional licensure—the latter making the institution responsible for credentialing of personnel under one overall state license. The nursing profession was almost unanimous in its opposition to the concept; however, it recognized some of the problems inherent in the current system of individual licensure, such as: lack of guarantee that the licensed nurse would not become obsolete in knowledge and practice; rigidity of curricula for the education of nurses; restrictive membership of many licensing boards; barriers to upward mobility; and, in some cases, interstate mobility. By the mid-seventies the profession was not only discussing mandatory continuing education for relicensure as a means of preventing obsolescence and incorporating new knowledge, but in some states laws to this effect were being seriously considered. In one state such a law has already been passed.

Nursing was expanding its scope of education, responsibility, and accountability. The legal implications of extending and expanding the practice of professional nursing were of real concern. In states across the country, nurses, along with other health workers and legal counsel, studied nurse practice acts. By the mid-seventies, preparation for changes was gaining momentum. Changes were being proposed in a variety of ways, such as current nurse practice acts, rewritten and expanded nurse practice acts, and/or additional amendments.

The situation in nursing education was unclear in the fifties, and the great majority of nurses continued to be prepared in diploma programs. Although the number of baccalaureate programs was increasing steadily, many of these were not truly baccalaureate programs since they did not include an upper division nursing major. The number of graduates remained small. Associate of Arts programs, on the other hand, increased more rapidly, and the growth of practical nurse programs was phenomenal—increasing from 71 programs in 1948 to 479 in 1957. There was considerable disagreement and misunderstanding about the direction nursing should take toward true professionalism. Part of the problem was due to the small numbers of nurses prepared at the master's level, and the fact that the majority of faculty and nursing leaders were themselves diploma graduates.

Nursing and nursing education was going through a revolution. There was widespread interest in nursing and nursing education among health professionals, general educators, and the general public, as well as nursing leaders. Nursing was planning and collaborating with others on a broad base in an attempt to meet the needs of society. It became part of the Southern Regional Education Board early in the fifties: soon after, it joined the Western Regional Board of Higher Education, and, somewhat later, the New England Board of Higher Education.

The soul-searching work of seeking answers to questions about changing goals and purposes of nursing and nursing education was well under way. Some of the unresolved problems were: What should the role and responsibilities of the nurse be in relation to other health professionals? How should nurses be educated? Why had the graduates of baccalaureate programs not made more impact on nursing practice?

Should nursing prepare more generalists or more specialists, in light of the knowledge and technology explosion? How could nursing attract more young people to enter the profession? Nursing struggled to find answers to these and many other questions.

Spurred by monies appropriated by the National Mental Health Act, psychiatric nursing took leadership in integrating psychiatric nursing concepts into baccalaureate nursing programs, and in developing graduate programs for the preparation of specialists in psychiatric nursing. Federal support through traineeships was soon available for the preparation of administrators, supervisors, and teachers in all areas, and for beginning practitioners in public health nursing.

The need for research in nursing was becoming increasingly evident. In 1952, the first issue of *Nursing Research* was published, and in 1955, the first federal money to be earmarked specifically for nursing research became available. As the recognition of the need for research and the development of a firm theoretic base in nursing became increasingly evident, educational preparation at the doctoral level for nurses became both a necessity and a reality.

Rapid changes and developments in nursing and nursing education during the sixties were inevitable and imperative. Society wanted and expected more and better health care. College education was demanded by more and more people, and a bachelor's degree was generally accepted as a base for the professions. The pool of potential candidates for baccalaureate nursing education had increased markedly as a result of the postwar baby boom. Scientific and technologic advances and research had resulted in a tremendous increase in knowledge relative to medicine and health. All these factors converged to support the belief, long held by many educators and leaders in nursing, that nursing, in a manner similar to other professions, must prepare its practitioners within institutions of higher education. The American Nurses' Association took leadership in clarifying this stand when in 1965 it issued the historic Position Paper on Education for Nursing. Its main components were:

1. Education for those who work in nursing should take place in institutions of learning within the general education system.
2. The education for all those who are licensed to practice nursing should take place in institutions of higher education.
3. Minimum preparation for beginning professional nursing practice should be baccalaureate degree education in nursing.
4. Minimum preparation for beginning technical nursing practice at the present time should be associate degree education in nursing.
5. Education for assistants in the health service occupations should be intensive preservice programs in vocational education institutions rather than on-the-job training programs.[25]

Shortly thereafter, the National League for Nursing supported the trend toward college-based programs of nursing. It recommended an orderly movement of nursing education toward institutions of higher learning in such a way that the flow of nurses into the community not be interrupted. There were and continue to be many within nursing who neither agree with nor support the American Nurses' Association position, and the struggle within nursing between those advocating either diploma or baccalaureate education as the base for nursing has continued to be a bitter one—far from resolved by the end of the sixties.

During this period the American Nurses' Association grew in political maturity and began to use its enormous influence to initiate, support, and endorse sound federal legislation. Its concern for human dignity was shown in its early leadership in admitting all nurses to membership regardless of race, creed, or color. When a national health insurance plan under the Social Security Administration was proposed, the American Nurses' Association publicly supported the plan in spite of opposition to it by the American Medical Association and the American Hospital Association.

Care of the patient had always been the primary focus of nursing. There was a growing concern, however, about whether nursing was continuing to maintain this responsibility. Increased use of the fruits of technology, such as computers, was resulting in depersonalization of care. Increasing numbers of paraprofessionals and other ancillary workers were participating in direct patient care. Nursing felt a renewed need to give highest priority to clinical practice. The desire for greater clinical expertise resulted in the development of graduate programs to prepare clinical specialists in such areas as maternity and child nursing, medical and surgical nursing, psychiatric nursing, rehabilitation nursing, and community health nursing. In addition, a whole variety of short, technical, nondegree courses were established to prepare nurses for expanded roles, such as the pediatric nurse practitioner. The need for specialists in nursing to contribute to comprehensive care had been well accepted. By the seventies, nurse specialists and pracitioners were increasing, both in variety and in numbers.

Until recent years, research about nursing had lagged somewhat behind that of other professions. Much of the early research concerned itself with studies of the occupation of nursing and its administration and teaching aspects, rather than with scientific investigation into its nursing practice. As the number of nurses prepared at the doctoral level increased in the sixties, the content and quality of nursing research improved markedly. Emphasis was placed on the development of nursing theory and on scholarship in nursing, through writing as well as research.

The pattern of nursing education continued to change in the seventies. Table 1 shows the number of state-approved nursing programs which prepared students for beginning practice in nursing for each one-year period from 1970 through 1974. The greatest increase was in the number of associate degree programs, with a steady decline in the number of diploma programs. The major contribution to growth was in the practical or vocational nursing programs.

The general picture in relation to master's and doctoral programs in nursing was one of modest growth, as shown in Table 2.

Nursing was plagued by persistent problems relating to manpower supply and demand, roles and functions, diverse patterns of nursing education, and career conflicts. Although these problems were within the profession of nursing itself, there was need for a broadly representative group to study and analyze them objectively in relation to the overall needs of society. A National Commission for the Study of Nursing Education[26] came into being as a result of the growing concern on the part of nursing, nursing organizations, and society in general about ways to improve the delivery of health care to the American people. The commission started its work in 1967, financed by the American Nurses' Association, the National League for Nursing, the American Nurses' Foundation, the Avalon Foundation, the Kellogg Foundation, and a most generous anonymous benefactor.

Basically, the study focused on supply of and demand for nurses, nurses' roles and functions, nursing education, and nursing careers.

The first summary report and recommendations of the National Commission on Nursing and Nursing Education, commonly referred to as the Lysaught Report, appeared in the February 1970 issue of the *American Journal of Nursing*. The report set basic priorities for three needed changes in nursing practice and education. These were:

1. Increased research into both the practice of nursing and the education of nurses;

TABLE 1. Number of Programs Which Prepare for Beginning Practice in Nursing, as of October 15, for the Years 1970 Through 1974.*

ACADEMIC YEAR	ASSOCIATE DEGREE	DIPLOMA	BACCA-LAUREATE	TOTAL BASIC RN PROGRAM	PRACTICAL OR VOCATIONAL	GRAND TOTAL
1970	444	641	270	1,355	1,253	2,608
1971	491	587	285	1,363	1,291	2,654
1972	541	543	293	1,377	1,310	2,687
1973	574	494	305	1,373	1,306	2,679
1974	598	461	313	1,372	1,315	2,687

**National League for Nursing, "Educational Preparation for Nursing, 1974."* Nursing Outlook *23 (September 1975):8.*

TABLE 2. Enrollments in Nursing Programs Leading to Masters and Doctoral Degrees* with Percentage of Enrollments Which are Full Time, 1970–74.†

AS OF OCT. 15	MASTER'S PROGRAMS			DOCTORAL PROGRAMS		
	Total	Full Time	Percent Full Time	Total	Full Time	Percent Full Time
1970	4,765	3,529	74.1	312	120	38.5
1971	5,405	3,925	72.6	293	151	41.1
1972	6,342	4,324	68.1	402	180	44.8
1973	6,786	4,159	61.2	375	161	42.9
1974	7,924	4,462	56.3	482	192	39.8

**Pertains only to 9 doctoral programs in nursing education departments or divisions. Excludes R.N.'s taking doctorates in other departments or disciplines.*

†National League for Nursing, "Educational Preparation for Nursing," 1974. Nursing Outlook 23 *(September 1975):8.*

2. Enhanced educational systems and curricula based on the results of that research; and
3. Increased financial support for nurses and for nursing to ensure adequate career opportunities that will attract and retain the number of individuals required for quality health care in the coming years.[27]

The report, published in 1970 in *Abstract for Action,* sparked discussion and controversy. Determination of the Commission to begin implementation of the recommendations resulted in additional financial support for three more years. In 1973, the publication *From Abstract Into Action* reported progress. By the mid-seventies, it was hard to evaluate the impact of this study. The National Joint Practice Commission had been formed. Several state master planning committees had developed. Some diploma schools had closed, and a few had begun to grant degrees. In addition, the National Commission for the Study of Nursing and Nursing Education had made several recommendations:

1. Development of a greater knowledge base by increased research into the practice of nursing and education of nurses
2. Improved educational systems and curricula based on the results of that research
3. Clarification of roles and practices conjointly with other health professionals to ensure the delivery of optimum care
4. Increased financial support for nurses and for nursing to ensure adequate career opportunities that will attract and retain the number of individuals required for quality health care in the coming years[28]

PUBLIC HEALTH NURSING

In spite of its hardships, the depression did a great deal to stimulate the development of public health and public health nursing. Many volunteered to help relieve the suffering of others. A large number of these volunteers worked with public health nurses. For many it was their first acquaintance with public health nursing, and they became strong advocates in publicizing the services of public health nurses and in recruiting others for this work.

Relief projects of all kinds were financed by the federal government, with each state assuming responsibility for their implementation. Several thousand nurses were employed in these projects, and for many it was their introduction to public health nursing. In order to utilize those nurses effectively, it was necessary for the federal government to provide consultation services to the states. In 1934, Pearl McIver became the first public health nurse employed by the United States Public Health Service to provide consultation services to state health departments. At this time only a few state health departments included public health nursing in their budgets. Two years later all the states had budgeted funds for some kind of public health nursing consultative services.

The need to collaborate with others in meeting people's health needs had long been a principle of public health nursing, but the depression and its aftereffects brought this need into sharp focus. The collaboration of health professionals to solve common problems became fairly frequent.

The Social Security Act, passed in 1935, was designed to alleviate some of the ravages of the depression. Title VI of this act was particularly related to public health programs and was the harbinger of a new relationship between the federal government and the states. The overall purpose was to stimulate a nationwide program of public health for the protection and promotion of the health of the people.

There were two major provisions in Title VI. One called for an annual appropriation of $8,000,000 to assist states, counties, and medical districts in establishing and maintaining adequate health services. Some of this money was also available for the training of public health workers. The other called for an annual appropriation of not more than $2,000,000 for research and the investigation of disease and problems of sanitation. Monies were made available on a matching basis to the states. The amount available to each state was based on population, financial need, and the existence of special health problems.

As a result of Title VI, existing public health nursing programs were expanded, and new ones were developed. The public health nurse became a familiar figure in many of the rural areas where she had been unknown before. These nurses for the most part were employed under the aegis of the existing county governmental unit. Bedside nursing care of the sick, which had previously been thought of as the responsibility of the voluntary visiting nurse association, became part of their services to families, in addition to the more traditional services of health guidance and promotion. At the same time, the maternal, child health, and crippled children's provisions of the Social Security Act were introducing public health nurses to families who previously had not known about their existence.

By 1940, the appropriation of funds under Title VI had tripled. The organization of state health departments had been strengthened; more than 4,000 health workers had received training in accredited schools; 970 additional counties had some full-time public health services; and 1,150 additional clinics had been established for the treatment of venereal disease.[29] For the first time the United States Public Health Service became a partner and advisor to the state health departments, and through them to the local communities.

Approximately 3,000 of the persons who received training funds were public health nurses. Public health nursing had been included as part of federal and state Civil Service Commissions, and 1 year of academic preparation had become accepted as preparation for public health nursing practice. By 1944, only accredited baccalaureate programs which included the equivalent of this public health nursing preparation were being approved. Continuing emphasis was placed on the social and public health aspects of health and illness as part of all good nursing. Qualified public health nurses were added to hospital nursing staffs and nursing school faculties. Increasingly, public health field experience was becoming an accepted requirement for all students in baccalaureate programs accredited for public health nursing.

The war, with its medical care program for military personnel and their dependents plus the massive health education programs directed toward the civilian population, contributed to the development of a health consciousness in the people which included the belief that good health care was a basic human right. In the years immediately following the war, chronic diseases and accidents became the leading causes of death; the infant death rate declined dramatically; life expectancy at birth increased to 67 years and over; new drugs and vaccines contributed to the control of communicable diseases; graduate schools of public health were established in several universities; the multidisciplinary teaching approach in the training of public health workers was widely acclaimed; the Hospital Survey and Construction Act was passed by Congress in 1946, and hospital utilization was expanding rapidly; the

United States had become a member of the World Health Organization; and American health professionals were participating in and contributing to the development of international health programs.

Debate over the issue of a compulsory national health insurance plan was continuous and gaining momentum as voluntary insurance plans of various kinds became available to the people. Rosen[30] states that by 1953, 59 percent of the civilian population was covered by some kind of hospital insurance. This was in contrast to 1933 when there was only one Blue Cross Hospital Service Plan with a total enrollment of 2,000. Medical group prepaid practice plans appeared and were challenged in the courts by the American Medical Association. A few hospital-based home care programs were developing. These plans made it possible for patients who had been discharged from the hospital to their own homes to have all professional and therapeutic services available to them. The Montefiore Home Care Program was one of the earliest plans and provided a model for further developments. The Montefiore Plan contracted with the New York Visiting Nursing Service for nursing care. A few visiting nurse associations were experimenting with a prepayment plan for nursing service, but these efforts did not succeed, partly because of a lack of an actuarial base. Blue Cross was beginning to set up some experiments in the early discharge of patients from the hospital in order to determine the cost of including public health nursing as one of the benefits for Blue Cross members. At the same time, the Metropolitan Life Insurance and John Hancock Life Insurance companies discontinued their home nursing programs that had been started in the early part of the century. The need for a health care system for all Americans was becoming increasingly obvious and urgent. There was tacit acceptance of the fact that medical care was a right for everyone and not just a privilege for those who could afford it. The questions remained about how it should be delivered, how it should be paid for, and how it should be fashioned.

In the late forties and early fifties public health and public health nursing seemed to be imbued with a concern for how services should be organized and administered. There was a feeling that if the services were organized similarly in each community throughout the country, the people could get the services they needed. It was generally accepted that each community should have a full-time health department. Vital statistics, control of communicable diseases, environmental sanitation, laboratory services, maternal and child health services, and health education under the aegis of the health department were the touchstones of this effort. It was considered that an area should have at least 50,000 people in order to establish and support an efficient health department. In 1946 a committee of representatives from all federal and national agencies interested in public health nursing issued a statement which said in part that one public health nurse should combine both bedside nursing care and health guidance to the entire family. Organizational patterns were recommended for the communities according to population size. Three patterns were recommended:

1. All public health nursing service, including care of the sick at home, administered and supported by the health department. This is the most satisfactory pattern for rural communities.
2. Preventive services carried by the health department, with one voluntary agency working in close coordination with the health department, carrying responsibility for bedside nursing and some special fields. At present this type of organization is the most usual one in large cities.
3. A combination service jointly administered and jointly financed by official and voluntary agencies with all field service rendered by a single group of public health nurses. Such a combination of services is most desirable in smaller cities because it provides more and better service for each family.[31]

There was general agreement that there should be one public health nurse for each unit of 2,500 people if bedside nursing service was included. One public health nurse to each unit of 5,000 persons was adequate if bedside nursing was not part of the services offered.

Thus, the model was developed. There was a feeling that if somehow it could be adhered to, the public health nursing needs of people would be met. One of the earlier premises of public health nursing, which stressed that each community must define its own health needs and determine how best to organize to meet its needs, seemed to have been forgotten during this period of preoccupation with the organizational patterns of public health and public health nursing.

It was during this time that the initiative and the leadership role of public health nurses diminished, and public health nursing entered a period in which it was constantly defending its role and responsibility in the community as well as its contribution to nursing. It seemed to be striving to establish a beachhead in which its position would be clear, as evidenced by the concentration on the development of organizational patterns that should be followed by each community. In the process the many forces in society that were operating to make the patterns obsolete before they could become operational were ignored.

Strides were being made in nursing education, with baccalaureate programs developed in several colleges and universities. The programs were geared both for the high school graduate and for the registered nurse who was a graduate of a diploma program in nursing. The underlying aim in the development of the baccalaureate programs was that the graduates be prepared for the beginning practice of nursing in any area, including public health nursing. Much of the content which previously had been considered preparation exclusively for public health nursing was now deemed necessary for all graduates of a baccalaureate program and was integrated throughout the curriculum. The community was discovered as a laboratory for nursing students, and nursing educators were clamoring for all kinds of community experiences for their students. Thus, almost overnight, public health nursing was stripped of its content and of the setting in which it functioned. Separate elaborate accreditation procedures were set up for the public health and public health nursing component in baccalaureate programs. This development was no doubt partly due to the need for public health nursing to retain and defend its position in the rapidly changing educational scene.

By the early sixties, public health and public health nursing began to emerge from their defensive cocoon and to become more aware of the society of which they were a part. Separate accreditation procedures were abolished, and theory and practice in public health nursing became a requirement for all baccalaureate programs in nursing. In 1964, the American Nurses' Association defined a public health nurse as a graduate from a baccalaureate program in nursing accredited by the National League for Nursing.

The contribution of public health and public health nursing to the solution of the nation's health problems was less clear than it had been at the beginning of the period. In spite of the fact that there was a larger pool of nurses who were prepared in public health nursing, the numbers of public health nurses were not increasing—in fact, proportionately, there was a decrease. There were still many communities without any public health nursing service available; on the other hand, there were many with two, three, or more agencies providing public health nursing with many gaps and duplications. More and more professional, semiprofessional, and indigenous community workers were appearing and further complicating the picture. The existing public health and public health nursing agencies were having difficulty in adjusting to new workers and new programs. Combination services had not expanded as had been anticipated.

At the same time many areas did not have any full-time public health services, and many of the health departments which had been well established were not responsive to the changing needs of the people. The cost of medical care was rising steadily, but the opposition of the American Medical Association to a federally sponsored health insurance plan was becoming more and more adamant. Congress was appropriating more funds each year for specific diseases rather than for general public health programs; voluntary agencies had multiplied, and often disproportionate amounts of money were contributed for diseases or conditions that were not particularly significant to the overall health of the people. New health workers, both professional and nonprofessional, were constantly emerging, with much overlapping and duplication of responsibilities; and health facilities of all kinds appeared with no coordination or planning for comprehensive delivery of health services to all the people.

New health problems demand new solutions. The role of health departments and of public health in general in the solution of these problems was unclear. The problems of the nuclear age with its attendant radiologic health hazards were mainly unsolved. Noise abatement, smog, water pollution, overcrowding, chronic illness, a rising infant death rate with only a slight increase in life expectancy, accidents, overpopulation, premature deaths—particularly in the young adult male—were some of the health problems to be tackled in the immediate future. The concept of the "community of solution," in which health problems and their solutions superseded political jurisdiction, was beginning to emerge as a method of approach.

On the brighter side, some exciting community health demonstrations were in progress, and public health nurses were becoming involved increasingly in a colleague relationship with multidisciplinary teams in providing new and comprehensive services for groups of patients and families. There was a trend toward developing community health programs based on the needs of the community rather than on the services offered by a particular agency. Federal legislation, such as the laws pertaining to Medicare and the certification of Home Health Agencies, the health component of model cities' programs, poverty programs with their emphasis on neighborhood health centers and citizen participation, comprehensive health planning, and the National Health Planning and Resources Act of 1974 were pinpointing the need for a clearer definition of public health nursing and a delineation of the competencies of public health nurses. In 1966, the American Public Health Association and the National League for Nursing jointly launched a program for the accreditation of community health nursing services. This was the first effort to apply the accreditation process to the delivery of nursing service.

By the mid-seventies, public health nurses were employed in a variety of settings, such as hospitals, home care programs, mental health centers, housing developments for the elderly, and ambulatory services. Graduate programs for the preparation of specialists in public health nursing had been developed and some of these were including practitioner preparation. Public health nurses were working collaboratively with specialists in other areas of nursing to meet the nursing needs of people wherever they were found. Comprehensive health service was becoming the major theme, with emphasis on the needs of the individual, the family, and the community, and on how the needs could be met with the available resources. The road ahead was unclear, but the period of introspection and defensiveness of public health nursing was ending and a new era was beginning. In this new era public health nursing would be in full partnership with other specialists in nursing and with allied health professionals in providing comprehensive health care to the people.

SUMMARY

There are no key or universal words to characterize the years in America between the New Deal and the mid-seventies; affluence, enlightenment, apathy, depression, soul-searching, involvement, and social revolution might each be descriptively applicable. The New Deal had a catalytic effect—making it possible for the country to pull itself out of the depression, and heralding the centralization of the federal government.

The impact of war on any society is always cataclysmic, and World War II was no exception. The people and the economy mobilized and were able once again to convert their resources for the gigantic war effort. The postwar period, in spite of problems of economic readjustment from war to so-called peace, produced economic progress for a while, and there was a feeling of optimism combined with a certain complacency about the present and the future of the country. Some of the pervading ideas were:

1. America was still a land of opportunity and the future was bright.
2. The nuclear family was the prototype of the American family.
3. Mobility was a way of life.
4. The suburbs were increasingly desirable as a place to live.
5. Science and technology could solve all problems.
6. Answers to almost anything could be found through research.
7. Government and private industry must form a partnership.
8. Education was necessary so that people could understand what was going on.
9. Quality health care was a right for all.
10. The federal government was responsible for the welfare of the people.

Between the sixties and mid-seventies a marked change occurred in the outlook of the country. Many of the insistent concerns of the times seemed to converge into a growing revolution of values. Major concerns were: the civil rights movement, which stood at the heart of social consciousness; the New Frontier and Great Society of the Kennedy and Johnson eras, with their impact on rising expectations of the people; the emphasis on large-scale planning with increasing federal legislation and involvement; and the legal definition of poverty for the first time. Fears and questions about the future were raised—about our continued, increasing involvement in the Vietnam War, about the military stance and power of the federal government, about the priority of war over peace at a time of expanding domestic problem, and about corruption at the very heart of the government, triggered by Watergate. Pessimism was increasing, and questions were being raised about the basic values and quality of life itself. The youth of the country were particularly concerned. There was a growing feeling that people must be actively involved in making decisions which affect them; that equality of opportunity must become a reality, not just a slogan; and that educational programs are irrelevant for today's world and must be reorganized. The cities were deteriorating, the population was increasing, and air pollution, crime, and delinquency were growing problems. Science and technology were getting out of hand and resulting in depersonalization. Disenchantment with the status quo was spreading. The need for action on social issues was imperative.

Perhaps it was destiny that gave nursing the ability and strength to survive the depression, the Second World War, and the stressful and dynamic years that followed. Buffeted and influenced by diverse and wide-ranging social forces, nursing was able to respond, mature, and in its own right directly influence the quality of life of the American people.

At the beginning of the period nursing still was hampered by the "angel of mercy" and "handmaiden of the physician" images, and by the apprenticeship system of education. By the end of the sixties the independent functions of nursing had been identified, nursing was firmly entrenched in institutions of higher learning, baccalaureate nursing education had been accepted by the professional nursing organization as the minimum requirement for entrance into the profession, and the master's degree in nursing was accepted as preparation for advanced practice. Doctoral programs in nursing had been established, and nursing research was contributing to the development of a theoretic base for professional nursing practice. Colleague relationships had been established with professional and citizen groups concerned with improvement of the overall health care delivery system. Nurses had developed in political know-how and expertise and were actively involved in bringing about change.

Gigantic changes occurred during this whole period, and there were certain times in which nursing had to make crucial decisions—each of which affected its future directions. These times were the depression and its aftermath, the Second World War, the postwar period of readjustment, and the social revolution of the sixties. As an outgrowth of the depression, the decision was made that graduate nurses, rather than students, should provide direct service to patients in the hospital. Thus, the focus shifted from private duty nurses giving care in the home, to staff nurses giving care in the hospital. At the start of World War II opportunities for nurses had increased, more nurses had had direct patient-care experience in the hospital, and nursing was in a good position to contribute more fully to the direct care of military personnel and their dependents all over the world. Nurses were given full officer status, making it possible for them to contribute on an equal basis with others of similar rank.

By the end of the war nursing had become much more aware of the society of which it was a part, and was better able to respond directly to the forces and needs of the broader community. Large numbers of nurses took advantage of the G.I. Bill and enrolled in institutions of higher learning. This growing pool of nurses with broader education gave added impetus to the need for moving nursing into the mainstream of higher education—long a vision of some nursing leaders. At the same time, the level of education of all the people had risen, great strides were being made in science and technology, and the people were demanding more comprehensive health care. The American Nurses' Association, with a better-educated membership, took leadership as the spokesman for organized nursing. It took stands on national issues, supporting legislation on nursing and health matters and taking a positive stand for national health insurance—a position opposite to that of the American Medical Association. It was one of the first professional organizations to open its membership to all nurses regardless of race, color, or creed at a time when many state nurses' associations had membership restrictions. An economic security program for the improvement of working conditions and salaries of nurses also came under its aegis. It was largely due to the efforts of the American Nurses' Association and its growing political acumen that federal legislation was passed for the support of higher education in nursing and nursing research. A further indication of the nation's recognition of nursing as a profession was the establishment of the Division of Nursing as a permanent part of the United States Public Health Service.

At the same time there was much furor and dissension among nurses, with continual debate about how nurses should be educated. In spite of the position of the American Nurses' Association that all nursing education should be under the umbrella of educational institutions, the rank and file of nurses were not completely sold on the idea.

The changes in nursing and its progress toward professionalism occurred at differing rates for institutional nursing and public health nursing. Prior to World War II public health nursing was the unofficial leader in nursing education and nursing practice. In the postwar years, however, this leadership was taken over by the nursing educators. Public health nursing seemed to have lost its ability to respond to the forces in society that were reshaping the education and practice of all professionals. Its reaction was one of hanging on to proven practices and retaining the status quo. The partnership of public health nursing with public health was by this time firmly entrenched and mutually beneficial. One of the side effects, however, was the difficulty experienced by many nurses in public health in clarifying whether their primary identity was to nursing or to public health. Public health nursing had taken on an aura of invincibility and had become rather complacent and smug about its leadership role in the education of public health nurses, in its working conditions and personnel policies, and in the scope of its practice. Therefore, it was not prepared for the fact that changes in nursing and nursing education would have a direct effect upon its leadership in these areas, and that the uniqueness of public health nursing was not defined by these peripheral elements.

The clamor by the people for health services that would meet their needs, the requests by educators and nursing practitioners for a clarification of the uniqueness of public health nursing, the changing role of government in the delivery of health care, and the increased educational level of the people seemed generally to be ignored by public health nursing, and rather elaborate procedures were set up to defend the status quo. Public health was also faced with the same dilemma, and it almost seemed as if public health nursing opted to identify more closely with public health and its problems than with nursing and its problems.

Increased hospital utilizations; growth of health insurance plans; application of new technology, drugs, and surgical procedures; and new kinds of health workers all contributed to the changing role of the hospital and drastically affected institutional nursing. Initial steps were taken to extend hospital services into the community with the development of home care programs and expanded ambulatory services. These developments were destined to bring institutional nursing and public health nursing closer together. By the mid-seventies, the emphasis was centered on comprehensive health care, and the competency with which people met this goal became more important than the setting in which the care was provided. Peer review and accountability were being stressed.

By the time of the social revolution of the sixties, nursing, in spite of its problems, had made great strides toward professionalism. It was able to identify more clearly its contribution to the health of the people; public health nursing had become an inherent component of all baccalaureate programs in nursing; and nursing was collaborating with the other professions in delivering health care, was developing colleague relationships with other disciplines, and was playing a partnership role with others in higher education. The necessity for higher education to improve nursing practice was generally accepted, and graduate programs emphasizing excellence in practice were developing. Nursing had become a force in itself and was in a position to influence the direction and quality of health care for the nation.

Medical care, just one aspect of health care, was a paradox in the mid-seventies. It could be characterized as being among the best in the world and also the poorest. It was in a state of transition. The impact of science, technology, and the use of computers on medical care was just beginning to be felt and was resulting in far-reaching changes in medicine itself as well as in its delivery. The frightening rise in the cost of medical care, the inequities in the availability and quality of care, and the appalling fragmentation of services were bringing into sharper focus what was perhaps the basic problem—the fact that there was no overall viable health care system. Left pretty much to its own devices, American medicine had developed into a multifaceted uncoordinated complex within which one could identify two different systems: one for the poor financed largely through public funds; and one for those who could still afford to meet the spiraling costs of private medical care. The financial burden of supporting this kind of program was becoming unbearable, particularly for the middle-class American, and there was a sense of urgency that something must be done soon to alleviate the situation. Care for both the rich and poor could be characterized as being crisis-oriented, fragmented, and plagued by problems resulting from maldistribution and poor utilization of manpower and resources.

The consumer was very much concerned about his care and was actively involved with other health workers in looking at both the needs of the people and the needs of the community, and demanding more control over how these needs might be met. The health team, formerly the doctor, the nurse, and the sanitarian, had expanded to include consumers and providers of care, as well as a growing number and variety of paraprofessional workers. This expanded team was attempting to design and develop new and better ways to bring health care to the people, particularly to those in the inner cities. Many of the approaches being tried were innovative and creative and were resulting in the lowering of some of the institutional barriers to change. Demonstration neighborhood health centers, multiservice centers, model cities health programs, satellite clinics, and store-front clinics were mushrooming. Prepaid group practice plans and health maintenance organizations were increasing.

The government had attempted, through multiple legislation, to encourage regional and comprehensive approaches to health care, with emphasis on planning and citizen involvement. Experience with Medicare and Medicaid had made increasingly evident the almost insurmountable cost of health care and the need for comprehensive planning. Solutions to new health problems, such as those relating to the environment and drug addiction, were being sought. Many people felt that the government should be more responsive to the country's health problems and place a higher priority on health. The pressure on the government to come up with some kind of overall national health plan was intensifying, and the debate over what kind of a plan it should be and how it should be financed continued. As might be expected, many special-interest and power groups were throwing their hats into the ring. The only area of real agreement seemed to be that there was need for some kind of national health plan.

Nurses continued to constitute the largest group of health professionals involved in patient care. In 1968 there were approximately 680,000 registered nurses employed full or part time in nursing.[32] Of this number, 50,492, or 7.4 percent, were employed in public health.[33]

The whole question of the role of the nurse and her place in the health-care system still remained unclear and was further complicated by rapid changes within the system itself. Direct application of the fruits of research and of technologic and scientific developments had resulted in dramatic changes in patient care. As a result many questions are being raised about the need for additional skill, knowledge, continuing education, and levels of responsibility for nurses as well as other health professionals. There was heightened concern over depersonalization of care resulting from increasing emphasis on computers and technologic equipment. People were concerned also over the fact that nursing had been so preoccupied with administrative and organizational activities that it had gradually abdicated to licensed practical nurses, aides, and other ancillary workers, as well as to machines, its responsibility for provision of direct patient care. Nursing, by the seventies, was giving greater priority to clinical practice, professional competence, and accountability. More and more research was clinically oriented and directed toward development of a firmer theoretic base for the practice of nursing and for improved quality of care. Emphasis on clinical practice had resulted in the development of increasing numbers of graduate programs designed to prepare clinical specialists and practitioners of all kinds.

The knowledge explosion, and resulting changes in medical care, had evidenced the need for a health worker prepared to assist the physician in a different way. Whether this should be a new kind of paraprofessional worker or a nurse with additional preparation was as yet unclear. Special programs to prepare nurses for expanded roles, such as the pediatric nurse practitioner and the maternity nurse practitioner, and other programs to prepare physicians' assistants and other paraprofessionals were developing willy nilly with very little clarification about legality, relationships to each other, or to the overall health system. There was renewed discussion of the career-ladder concept. There was a growing feeling that many questions about roles, responsibilities, and relationships must be answered in the 1970s and 1980s.

Nursing education continued to encompass preparation on a variety of levels—a fact which results in much confusion on the part of the general public, as well as within the profession itself, about what nursing really is. The long-standing and continuous controversy about what kind of educational preparation was best for nursing was heightened by the 1965 Statement on Professional Nursing by the American Nurses' Association. In 1968, it was estimated that 84.8 percent of nurses were prepared in diploma programs, and 1.8 percent in associate degree programs.[34] Associate degree programs had shown the greatest increase, with a growth rate of 40 percent from 1967 to 1969.[35] The marked growth in nursing education programs, which had its initial emphasis in the mid and late 1960s, had almost certainly reached its peak in the mid-1970s.[36] The growth rate in admissions to associate degree programs declined more sharply than the growth rate of admissions to diploma and baccalaureate programs. The potential for upward mobility was evidenced by the increasing numbers of R.N.'s graduated from baccalaureate programs. The number of graduates from master's programs increased 8 percent from 1972–73 to 1973–74, with an increase in the numbers of part-time students. The number of students enrolled in doctoral programs in nursing remains small.[37] Emphasis in higher education in nursing was being given to scholarship, publication, and research.

The cost of nursing education, particularly collegiate nursing education, was staggering. Many colleges and universities, particularly private institutions, were questioning their ability to support such expensive programs without additional federal funds. The federal government, which had assumed major responsibility for financial support for graduate students, was withdrawing, rather than increasing, funds for the support of higher education.

At the same time many questions were being raised about the future of public health nursing services, particularly the visiting nurse associations and local health department nursing programs. The costs of visiting nurse associations were rising rapidly and soon might become prohibitive. The case loads consisted primarily of persons who were sick, preventive services being the responsibility of health departments. On the other hand, some health departments were including bedside care of the sick as part of their program, and in some instances preventive services were given second priority.

The joint venture of the National League for Nursing and the American Public Health Association, started in 1966 for accreditation of community health nursing services, was well established. In 1974 the name of the program was changed to Accreditation of Home Health Agencies and Community Nursing Services. Ninety-three community health nursing services had been accredited.[38] The precedent had been established for the need of some form of accreditation for nursing services within institutions as well as in the community.

Federal legislation, which included the development of comprehensive health centers and health maintenance organizations, had helped to pinpoint the need for an overhaul of the community nursing care system. In many instances comprehensive health centers, home care programs, and health maintenance organizations had been established outside the existing community health nursing system. Undoubtedly, there were many reasons why this had occurred, but as the trend toward provision of comprehensive services in health centers was occurring, new roles were emerging for public health nurses, and existing agency programs were becoming part of the network of comprehensive community health services.

One of the basic principles of public health nursing is collaboration with other professional and community groups to meet the needs of patients and families. The development of comprehensive health centers and health maintenance organizations provided the opportunity for public health nurses to fully implement this principle, and to become full-fledged members of a multidiscipline health team. This was an age of specialization with many specialized health personnel, including clinical specialists in nursing, participating in the health care of people.

REFERENCES

1. F. R. Dulles, *The United States Since 1865* (Ann Arbor: University of Michigan Press, 1959), p. 514.

2. P. Montague and C. Montague, "How Much Are We Eating?" *Saturday Review*, February 6, 1971, p. 51.
3. F. Graham, *Since Silent Spring* (Greenwich, Conn.: Fawcett Publications, 1970), p. 76.
4. N. A. Rockefeller, *Our Environment Can Be Saved* (Garden City, N.Y.: Doubleday & Company, 1970), p. 140.
5. D. Bell, "The Post-Industrial Society," in E. Ginsberg, ed., *Technology and Social Change* (New York: Columbia University Press, 1964), Ch. 2, p. 45.
6. Cambridge Research Institute, *Trends Affecting the U.S. Health Care System* (Washington, D.C.: Superintendent of Documents, 1976), p. 1.
7. *Ibid.*, p. 2.
8. *Ibid.*, p. 59.
9. H. B. Allen, *The Federal Government and Education* (New York: McGraw-Hill Book Company, 1950), pp. 8–10.
10. M. Brick, *Form and Focus for the Junior College Movement* (New York: Bureau of Publications, Teachers College, Columbia University, 1964), pp. 24–24.
11. H. D. Babbidge, Jr., and R. Rosenzweig, *The Federal Interest in Higher Education* (New York: McGraw-Hill Book Company, 1962), p. 24.
12. W. C. DeVane, *Higher Education in Twentieth Century America* (Cambridge, Mass.: Harvard University Press, 1965), p. 2.
13. U.S. Department of Health, Education and Welfare, Report to the Congress, *Nurse Training* (Bethesda, Md.: DHEW Publication No. [HRA] 75–41, 1974).
14. L. Bryson, ed., *Facing the Future's Risks* (New York: Harper & Brothers, 1953), p. 193.
15. G. Mowry, *The Urban Nation 1920–1960* (New York: Hill & Wang, 1965), p. 207.
16. M. A. Newcomer, *Century of Higher Education for American Women* (New York: Harper & Brothers, 1959), p. 214.
17. K. Patricia Gross, "Women Want Equality in Higher Education," *Educational Horizons* 52 (Winter 1973–74):72.
18. L. L. King, "An Epitaph for LBJ," *Harper's*, April 1968, pp. 21–22.
19. C. B. T. Lee, *The Campus Scene: 1900–1970* (New York: David McKay Company, 1970), p. 175.
20. L. Dietz and A. R. Lehoxey, *History and Modern Nursing*, 2d ed. (Philadelphia: F. A. Davis Company, 1967), p. 158.
21. E. L. Brown, *Nursing for the Future* (New York: Russell Sage Foundation, 1948), p. 198.
22. *Ibid.*, p. 116.
23. M. L. Montag, *The Education of Nursing Technicians* (New York: G. P. Putnam's Sons, 1951), p. 146.
24. M. E. Newton, "National League for Nursing Accreditation: From Four Viewpoints," *Nursing Outlook* 14 (March 1966):52.
25. E. Fritz and M. Murphy, "An Analysis of Positions on Nursing Education," *Nursing Outlook* 14 (February 1966):20.
26. National Commission for the Study of Nursing and Nursing Education, "Summary Report and Recommendations," *Amer. J. Nurs.* 70 (February 1970):286–93.
27. ———. "Summary Report and Recommendations," *Amer. J. Nurs.* 70 (February 1970):285.
28. Deanne B. Taylor and Onalee H. Johnson, *Systematic Nursing Assessment: A Step Toward Automation* (Washington, D.C.: Superintendent of Documents, 1974), pp. 11–12.

29. R. Williams, *The United States Public Health Service* (Bethesda, Md.: The Commissioned Officers Association of the United States Public Health Service, Box 5874, 1951), p. 156.
30. G. Rosen, *A History of Public Health* (New York, MD Publications, 1958), p. 461.
31. National Organization for Public Health Nursing, "Desirable Organization of Public Health Nursing for Family Service," *Public Health Nurs.* 38 (August 1946):388.
32. American Nurses' Association, *Facts About Nursing* (New York: American Nurses' Association, 1969), p. 9.
33. D. E. Roberts, V. K. Saba, and H. K. Allen, "Census of Nurses in Public Health," *Amer. J. Nurs.* 70 (November 1970):2394.
34. American Nurses' Association, *Facts About Nursing* (New York: American Nurses' Association, 1969), p. 9.
35. National League for Nursing, "Educational Preparation for Nursing—1969," *Nursing Outlook* 18 (September 1970):55.
36. ———. "Educational Preparation for Nursing—1974," *Nursing Outlook* 28 (September 1975):578.
37. *Ibid.*, p. 581.
38. "NLN Home Health Agencies and Community Nursing Services Accredited by NLN," *Amer. J. Public Health* no. 24 (April 1976) 254–55.

BIBLIOGRAPHY

Abrams, C. *The City Is the Frontier*, New York: Harper & Row, 1965

Adams, W. "The State of Higher Education: Myths and Realities." *Amer. Assoc. Univ. Prof. Bulletin* 60 (June 1974):119–25.

Allen, H. B. *The Federal Government and Education.* New York, McGraw-Hill Book Company, 1950.

American Nurses' Association. *Facts About Nursing 1974–75.* Kansas City, Missouri: American Nurses' Association, 1974.

———. *Facts About Nursing.* New York: American Nurses' Association, 1969.

Axt, R. J. *The Federal Government and Financing Higher Education*, New York: Columbia University Press, 1952.

Babbidge, H. D., Jr., and Rosezweig, R. M. *The Federal Interest in Higher Education.* New York: McGraw-Hill Book Company,1962.

Brick, M. *Form and Focus for the Junior College Movement.* New York: Bureau of Publications, Teachers College, Columbia University, 1964.

Brown, E. L. *Nursing for the Future.* New York: Russell Sage Foundation, 1948.

Bryson, L., ed. *Facing the Future's Risks.* New York: Harper and Brothers, 1953.

Cambridge Research Institute. *Trends Affecting the U.S. Health Care System.* Washington, D.C., 1976.

Davis, E. C. "Women in Non-traditional Roles: Hurdles, Challenges, Rewards." *Educational Horizons* 53 (Spring 1975):98–101.

DeVane, W. C. *Higher Education in Twentieth Century America.* Cambridge, Massachusetts: Harvard University Press, 1965.

Dulles, F. R. *The United States Since 1865.* Ann Arbor, Michigan: The University of Michigan Press, 1959.

Editorial, "Nursing research—January 1971." *Nurs. Res.* 20 (January—February 1971):3

Ellul, J. *The Technological Society.* New York: Alfred A. Knopf, 1964.

Fritz, E., and Murphy, M. "An Analysis of Positions on Nursing Education." *Nurs. Outlook* 14 (February 1966):20–24.

Ginsberg, E., ed. *Technology and Social Change.* New York: Columbia University Press, 1964.

Graham, F., Jr. *Since Silent Spring.* Greenwich, Connecticut: Fawcett Publications, 1970.

Green, C. M. *The Rise of Urban America.* New York, Harper & Row, 1965.

Griffin, J. G., and Griffin, J. K. *Jensen's History and Trends of Professional Nursing.* 6th ed. St. Louis: The C. V. Mosby Company, 1969.

Gross, E. P."Women Want Equality in Higher Education." *Educational Horizons* 52 (Winter 1973–74):72–75.

Haupt, A. "The Government's Subcommittee on Nursing." *Public Health Nurs.* 34 (March 1942):147–54.

———."Bottlenecks in Our War Nursing Program." *Amer. J. Public Health* 33:666–70.

Janeway, E. "Realizing Human Potential: Focus on Women." *Educational Horizons* 52 (Winter 1973–74):51–59.

Joint Committee of the National Organization for Public Health Nursing and the United States Public Health Service. *The Public Health Nursing Curriculum Guide.* Distributed by the National League for Nursing, 2 Park Avenue, New York, 1942.

King, L. L. "An Epitaph for LBJ." *Harper's* 336 (April 1968):14–22.

Lee, C. B. T. *The Campus Scene: 1900–1970.* New York: David McKay Company 1970.

McIver, P. "Developments under the United States Public Health Service." *Public Health Nurs.* 38 (September 1936):585–90.

———. "WPA Projects for Registered Nurses." *Amer. J. Nurs.,* 37 (January 1937):35–37.

Montag. M. L. *The Education of Nursing Technicians.* New York: G. P. Putnam's Sons, 1951.

Montague, P., and Montague, C. "Mercury: How Much Are We Eating?" *Saturday Review,* February 6, 1971, pp. 50–55.

Mowry, F. *The Urban Nation 1920–1960.* New York, Hill and Wang, 1965.

National Commission for the Study of Nursing and Nursing Education. "Summary Report and Recommendations." *Amer. J. Nurs.* 70 (February 1970):279–94.

National League for Nursing. "Educational Programs for Nursing." *Nurs. Outlook,* 18 (September 1970):52–57.

———. "Educational Preparation for Nursing—1974." *Nurs. Outlook* 23 (September 1975):578–82.

———. "Home Health Agencies and Community Nursing Services Accredited by the NLN–APHA, April 1976." *Nurs. Outlook* 24:254–55.

National Organization for Public Health Nursing. "Desirable Organization for Public Health Nursing for Family Service." *Public Health Nurs.* 38 (August 1946):387–89.

———. "Minimum Qualifications of Those Appointed to Positions in Public Health Nursing." *Public Health Nurs.* 28 (March 1936):172–75.

Newcomer, M. *A Century of Higher Education for American Women.* New York: Harper and Brothers, 1959.

Newton, M. E. "National League for Nursing Accreditation: From Four Viewpoints." *Nurs. Outlook* 14 (March 1966):48–54.

Proceedings of the Sixteenth Annual Transportation Conference: Salzberg Memorial Lecture, November 9, 1964. *Coordination of Services—Basis for an Improved National Transportation System.* Syracuse, New York: The Business Research Center, Syracuse University.

Reinsberg, M. *Growth and Change in Metropolitan Areas and Their Relation to Metropolitan Transportation.* Evanston, Illinois: The Transportation Center at University, 1961.

Roberts, E. E., Saba, F. K., Ellen, H. K. "Census of Nurses in Public Health." *Amer. J. Nurs.* 70 (November 1970):2394–99.

Roberts, M. *American Nursing.* New York: The Macmillan Company, 1954.

Rockefeller, N. A. *Our Environment Can be Saved.* Garden City, New York: Doubleday and Company, 1970.

Rosen, G. *A History of Public Health.* New York: MD Publications, 1958.

Taylor, D. B., and Johnson, O. H. *Systematic Nursing Assessment: A Step Toward Automation.* Washington, D.C.: Superintendent of Documents, 1974.

U.S. Bureau of Census.*Statistical Abstracts of the United States.* 90th ed. Washington, D.C.: Government Printing Office, 1969.

U.S. Department of Health, Education and Welfare, *Report to the Congress. Nurse Training 1974.* Bethesda, Maryland: DHEW Publication No. (HRA) 75–41. 1974.

von Bertalanffy, L. "The World of Science and the World of Value." In *Contemporary Readings in Organizational Behavior.* New York, McGraw-Hill Book Company, 1972, ppp 5–16.

Williams, R. *The United States Public Health Service.* Bethesda, Maryland: The Commissioned Officers Association of the United States Public Health Service, Box 5874, 1951.

Wilson, I. "How Our Values are Changing." In *Contemporary Readings in Organizational Behavior.* New York: McGraw-Hill Book Company, 1972, pp. 17–29.

CHAPTER 4

THE CONTEMPORARY SCENE

This book is replete with references to the health care scene—the arena in which nursing joins the myriad health care providers in carrying out its role and function. In spite of remarkable advances in science and technology, the crisis in health persists and continues to be plagued with such persistent problems as

1. Escalating costs
2. Crisis and illness orientation
3. Fragmentation of services
4. Lack of uniformity in delivery systems
5. Maldistribution of facilities and manpower
6. Rising consumer demands for service and participation
7. Increasing medical malpractice suits

Repeated legislative attempts have failed to bring about basic changes in these inherent problems. It is with this setting as background that we shall look at contemporary nursing and nursing education and discuss some of the ways in which nursing has been responding to society's health care needs. We shall view its progress and some of its accomplishments and persistent problems.

Many people feel that nursing, after a long and hard struggle, is finally maturing and gaining true professional stature, and that its future looks bright. Others are concerned about its very survival. Whatever its future at this time, nursing has done a lot of soul searching and reevaluation, has clarified many of its values and goals, and is more sure of the direction in which it is heading.

The rapid development and expansion of health services, coupled with proliferation of specialists of all kinds, has resulted in confusion. The patient is caught trying to find his way through this tortuous network. Patients and families desperately need someone to help them find where to turn, to support them during crises, to coordinate and mobilize the multiplicity of services and resources for them, and to speak in their behalf. While the medical profession has given little attention to prevention of disease and promotion of health, nursing is assigning a high priority to both of these areas.

Partly in response to this situation, the concept of primary care is very much in the forefront of nursing today. It includes three aspects: (1) the first contact with the patient; (2) continuity of care—particularly of health maintenance; and (3) coordination of care. It attempts to help people into and through the health care system in some orderly fashion, and focuses on positive health. This concept is being incorporated into programs of nursing education, and nurses, particularly community health nurses, are increasingly providing primary care.

Another way in which nursing is changing today is through expansion and extension of its roles and functions. The term "nurse practitioner" is used to describe graduates of programs through which nurses are educated to broaden their professional nursing functions, to incorporate new knowledge, skills, and responsibilities; and to attempt to better meet the needs of the public for improved health care.

Many kinds of practitioners are prepared today. The literature is filled with descriptions of programs which prepare pediatric nurse practitioners, maternity nurse practitioners, family nurse practitioners, and community health nurse practitioners, to name just a few. The term "nurse practitioner," though controversial, misunderstood, and even rejected, has "caught on" in nursing. Many feel that it is what nursing is all about—that it is an idea whose time has come. In any case, nurse practitioner programs, designed to prepare nurses for expanded roles of all kinds, are proliferating. To date, there are no universally accepted prerequisites, program requirements, or methods of evaluation. Practitioner programs for registered nurses run the gamut from short-term continuing-education programs to two-year programs on a graduate level. This diversity has been the source of much confusion. However, certain common denominators have emerged. The nurse practitioner cares for the patient in a variety of settings rather than working for the institution. She works both interdependently and independently, and is responsible and accountable for her own decisions—a situation not always possible within the hierarchical setting of many contemporary health care institutions. She has increased knowledge and competence in physical and psychosocial assessment. By integrating these with her own nursing ability, she is better able to collaborate with the physician, and to give better care to the patient.

Care is at the core of nursing, and quality health care demands clinical expertise and knowledge. Another way in which nursing is responding to the needs of the public, and extending its scope of knowledge and expertise, is by educating clinical specialists in graduate programs in nursing. The graduates are prepared to be skilled clinicians, and also teachers, consultants, and clinical researchers. The role of the clinical specialists is still not entirely clear. As is true with nurse practitioners, contemporary institutional constraints present barriers for professional independence. Many clinical specialists have carved out their own roles, however, and are demonstrating creative ways to provide quality care.

In 1973, the American Nurses' Association, long a supporter of high standards of practice, started a voluntary program of certification designed to recognize individual achievement and excellence in the practice of nursing. Certification signifies that the nurse recipient has met special and rigorous criteria for individual achievement and superior performance in nursing practice. This program provides recognition for excellence in practice and holds promise of being a credentialing mechanism for competence.

The expansion and extension of the scope and functions of nursing has raised a gamut of questions and issues relating to territorial rights between medicine and nursing, and, ultimately, to the whole question of nurse practice acts. This has forced nursing to study and redefine nursing practice in light of the contemporary situation. Nurse practice acts in relation to both statutory law and common law are being studied. Statutory law refers to laws enacted by the legislative branch of the government, and common law has to do with the body of precedent developed by the courts over a long period of time. Common law is particularly important in the interpretation of practice acts for both medicine and nursing today. It reflects many of the changes in nursing practice which have been brought about by changes within the whole contemporary social and health setting.

One of the major areas of concern is the fact that expanded functions of nursing may infringe on functions which traditionally and clearly have fallen within the province of medicine. The whole question of whether the nurse practitioner should become an arm of medicine had to be dealt with. Fortunately, this has been settled—the nurse practitioner will remain a part of professional nursing.

State nurses' associations are actively involved in reviewing and rewriting nurse practice acts, or preparing additional amendments to acts for legislative considerations. Laws permitting nurses to carry out broader functions, and/or to practice independently, have been passed in some states and are being developed in others. These changes are being made state by state. The implied questions for this development are many—for example, how will this affect state licensure, the mobility of nurses, and so forth? Nursing has entered an exciting new era of expanded practice. It also has much to do to put its house in order.

The purpose of licensure for the practice of nursing is to protect the public. Licensure means that the nurse has met the legal requirements for the safe practice of nursing. The fact that new knowledge has grown at such a phenomenal rate has raised questions about how the nursing profession can guarantee that all its practitioners will keep their knowledge base up to date, and that nursing service will incorporate and reflect these changes. A commitment to lifelong learning, although an inherent part of nursing, is difficult to actualize universally, and even harder to guarantee for over one million registered nurses. Concern about prvention of obsolescence and the necessity for nursing to keep abreast of new knowledge has resulted in a resurgence of interest in and availability of a variety of short- and long-term continuing education programs. There has been confusion about the differences between advanced education, in-service education, and continuing education. The National Commission for the Study of Nursing and Nursing Education developed three definitions for the purpose of distinction. These are:

1. Advanced education: Sequence of professional courses aimed at developing specialized qualifications characterized by formal academic recognition of completion, such as the awarding of an advanced degree.
2. Continuing education: formalized learning experience or sequence designed to enlarge the knowledge or skills of practitioners. As distinct from advanced education, continuing education courses tend to be more specific, of generally shorter duration, and may result in certification of completion, or specialization, but not formal degrees.
3. In-service education: Programs administered by an employer designed to upgrade the knowledge and skills of employees for their functioning in that agency.[1]

The whole question of whether continuing education should be mandatory for relicensure is a subject for debate. In the belief that it is the responsibility of the profession to upgrade and control its practice, the American Nurses' Association is attempting to stimulate nurses to continue their educations on a voluntary basis. In contrast, the National League for Nursing supports the goal of continuing education for licensure renewal—with carefully planned implementation. While the pros and cons of these differing approaches are being debated, nurses in increasing numbers are enrolling in continuing education of all kinds and collecting continuing education units (CEUs). A continuing education unit is defined as the unit designated for ten hours of study in an approved continuing education program. Mechanisms for approval of programs are being established by each state nurses' association, while the American Nurses' Association has developed a computerized system by which information about the continuing education units of each nurse can be made readily available and transmittable.

Expanded functions, broadened knowledge base, legal sanctions for more independent judgments and decision-making responsibility—all of these and more make it imperative that nursing be accountable for its actions. The call for accountability is being sounded throughout the health care field, and consumers and third-party payers, as well as governmental and nongovernmental groups, are scrutinizing methods being used for the evaluation of services. Nursing must be accountable to its recipients in relation to: the value of the nursing service provided; the quality of the care; and the outcomes and costs. Efforts are being made to develop guidelines to insure this kind of accountability.

The American Nurses' Association has been the first, and so far the only professional organization to develop standards of practice for its members. On the basis of these Standards of Practice, each Division of Practice within the American Nurses' Association developed standards specific to its own area of specialization. Steps are being carried out for implementation of the Standards through regional workshops across the country. The purpose of the workshops is to help nurses understand the importance of the standards in relation to nursing practice, and how they can be implemented. Increasingly, programs of nursing education are using the standards as the basis for their curricula. The standards must be put into practice before their effectiveness can be evaluated. The implications for their application, not only for the improvement of nursing practice,but ultimately for health care, are many—for both the immediate and the distant future.

Nursing holds within its grasp the ability to be a vital political force in helping to shape the kind of health care system which will meet the needs of the people. It is increasingly involved in political action, using its professional expertise to initiate legislation, to evaluate legislation developed by others, and to provide initial input into the shaping of programs. There are those who think that nursing must become more involved in the decision-making process, or that it will have to put up with decisions made by others, and thus may be legislated out of existence. Fortunately, recognition of the need for political involvement has caught on and has been growing. Organized nursing, at the national level, has been involved with legislation for a long time. Activity at the state level is also on the move. In 1973, the American Nurses' Association announced the formation of a new political action unit—Nurses Coalition for Action in Politics (N-CAP). This grew out of an idea sparked by a national group—Nurses for Political Action (NPA). The whole movement for women's rights and the Equal Rights Amendment (ERA), perhaps destined to become the twenty-seventh amendment to the Constitution, lends support to the cause of nursing, still predominantly a women's profession. One of nursing's major challenges today is its need for current leadership and risk-taking in the political arena. The risks of inactivity and noninvolvement are too great to leave to chance. Economic security, including access to collective bargaining, has been an important part of the professional organizations. Nursing is no exception. The American Nurses' Association, one of whose major purposes is the welfare of nurses, has for some time been actively involved in providing and supporting an economic security program which is administered by each state. A recent amendment to the Taft-Hartley Act, barring active participation by supervisors in collective bargaining, has been of real concern to nursing, as only part of the responsibilities of nursing supervisors are managerial. The American Nurses' Assiation is encouraging the National Labor Relations Board to differentiate between professional organizations and labor unions for the purpose of collective bargaining. Resolution of this problem is still unclear.

During the past few years, many other national nursing organizations besides the American Nurses' Association have developed to meet the individual needs of nurses working in specialized clinical areas. The American Nurses' Association has provided leadership in organizing the Federation of Nursing Specialty Organizations and the ANA. The Federation meets periodically and discusses problems of common concern. This coordination of effort has helped in the avoidance of duplication and has aided in the identification of shared problems. One positive outcome is cooperation and improvement in communication, and increased understanding of the issues common to all of the nursing groups. Proliferation of nursing organizations is of real concern. At the June 1976 meeting of the Council of Baccalaureate and Higher Degree Programs of the National League for Nursing, the membership requested of the Board of Directors "that immediate action be taken to initiate a study in collaboration with other national nursing organizations of the existing national organizational structure of nursing with the purpose of evaluating to what extent it does and does not support the purposes of the nursing profession in relation to the health needs of society."[2]

The distribution of nurses and nursing expertise, in providing quality care across the country, is one of the critical issues which nursing faces today. In 1974, the estimated number of registered nurses was 857,000. Of these, 608,000 were employed full time and 249,000 were working on a part-time basis. The educational preparation was as follows: diploma program—75.7 percent; baccalaureate programs—15.2 percent; associate degree programs—6.7 percent; and master's and doctoral programs—3.3 percent.[3]

At present, 74 percent of active registered nurses are employed in hospitals, nursing homes, and other institutions. About 10 percent perform community health nursing functions as employees of public health agencies, home care programs, boards of education, and industry. About 12 percent are self employed, or work in physicians' offices, private organizations, or the federal government. The remaining 4 percent are faculty members and administrators on nursing education programs.[4]

The growing emphasis on health promotion and prevention of disease makes it imperative that nursing prepare its practitioners and distribute its expertise so that the country's changing health needs may be met. Many of these needs are in the family and the community.

REFERENCES

1. National Commission for the Study of Nursing and Nursing Education, *An Abstract for Action* (New York: McGraw-Hill Book Company, 1970).
2. "News and Reports," *Nursing Outlook* 24 (June 1976):340.
3. American Nurses' Association, *Facts About Nursing 74–75* (Kansas City, Mo.. American Nurses' Association, 1976), p. 3.
4. *Ibid.*, p. 5.

BIBLIOGRAPHY

American Nurses' Association. *Facts About Nursing 1974–75*. Kansas City, Missouri: American Nurses' Association, 1976.

———. *Standards for Nursing Practice*. Kansas City, Missouri: American Nurses' Association, 1973.

Anderson, W. M., Leonard, B. J., Yates, J. A. "Epigenesis of the Nurse Practitioner Role." *Amer. J. Nurs.* 74 (October 1974):1812–16.

Bullough, B. *The Law and the Expanding Nursing Role.* New York: Appleton-Century-Crofts, 1975.

Creighton, Helen. "The Malpractice Problem." In *The Nursing Clinics of North America.* 9. Philadelphia: W. B. Saunders Company, 1974, pp. 425–33.

DeAngelis, C., and Curran, W. J. "The Legal Implications of the Extended Roles of Professional Nurses." In *The Nursing Clinics of North America.* 9. Philadelphia: W. B. Saunders Company, 1974, pp. 403–10.

Dunkley, P. H. The ANA Certification Program. In *The Nursing Clinics of North America.* 9. Philadelphia: W. B. Saunders Company, 1974, p. 485–95.

Guy, J. S. "Institutional Licensure: A Dilemma for Nurses." In *The Nursing Clinics of North America.* 9. Philadelphia: W. B. Saunders Company, 1974, pp. 497–504.

Hinsvark, I. G. "Implications for Action in the Expanded Role of the Nurse." In *The Nursing Clinics of North America.* 9. Philadelphia: W. B. Saunders Company, 1974, pp. 411–23.

Kelly, L. Y. *Dimensions of Professional Nursing.* 3d edition. New York: The Macmillan Company, 1975.

Lambertson, E. C. "The Changing Role of Nursing and Its Regulation." In *The Nursing Clinics of North America.* 9. Philadelphia: W. B. Saunders Company, 1974, pp. 395–402.

McClure, M. "Quality Assurance and Nursing Education: A Nursing Service Director's View." *Nurs. Outlook* 24 (June 1976):367–69.

McMullen, D. "Accountability and Nursing Education." *Nurs. Outlook* 23 (August 1975):501–3.

Millard, R. "The New Accountability." *Nurs. Outlook* 23 (August 1975):496–500.

National Commission for the Study of Nursing and Nursing Education. *An Abstract for Action.* New York: McGraw-Hill Book Company, 1970.

"News and reports." *Nurs. Outlook* 24 (June 1976):340.

Ozimek, D. *The Nurse Practitioner: The Current Situation and Implications for Curriculum Change.* New York: National League for Nursing, 1976.

Stahl, A. G. "State Boards of Nursing: Legal Aspects." In *The Nursing Clinics of North America.* 9. Philadelphia: W. B. Saunders Company, 1974, pp. 505–12.

Stanton, M. "Political Action and Nursing." In *The Nursing Clinics of North America.* 9. Philadelphia: W. B. Saunders Company, 1974, pp. 579–85.

Trail, I. D. "The Legal Implications of Community Nursing Care. In *The Nursing Clinics of North America.* 9. Philadelphia: W. B. Saunders Company, 1974, pp. 453–57.

U.S. Department of Health, Education and Welfare. *Report to the Congress. Nurses Training, 1974.* Bethesda, Maryland: DHEW Publication No. (HRA) 75–41. 1974.

———. *Trends Affecting the U.S. Health Care System.* Bethesda, Maryland: DHEW Publication No. (HRA) 76–14503, October 1975.

Whitaker, J. G. "The Issue of Mandatory Continuing Education. In *The Nursing Clinics of North America.* 9. Philadelphia: W. B. Saunders Company, 1974, 457–483.

PART II
COMMUNITY HEALTH NURSING PROCESS

INTRODUCTION

In Part II we will look at the process by which the community health nurse carries out her responsibility to families and to communities. The process revolves around the nursing needs of families and communities, and the knowledge necessary to meet these needs. The term "public health nursing" has been replaced by the broader phrase "community health nursing." There are many meanings that can be given to this phrase; however, for the purpose of this book, the following definition has been developed:

Community health nursing is the field of nursing in which the family and community are the patients. Although it is concerned with the total health-illness spectrum, its primary focus is on the prevention of disease, and the promotion and maintenance of the highest level of health and well-being.

The Community health nurse works collaboratively with families and groups in identifying their health problems and nursing needs, in determining the nursing care plan, in mobilizing appropriate community resources, and in evaluating the nursing services given. She may provide the care herself or coordinate the services rendered by other members of the nursing and health team.

The community health nurse participates with professional and lay persons in identifying the factors within the community relevant to health. She collaborates in planning, implementing, and evaluating the community health program, and assumes leadership in interpreting nursing and defining nursing needs.

We believe community health nursing involves a process which includes five steps:

1. Determining and collecting pertinent information.
2. Analyzing the information to determine the health problems and identify the nursing needs.

3. Determining the nursing care plan.
4. Implementing the nursing care plan.
5. Evaluating the nursing care plan.

This process is equally applicable to the individual, the family, or the community. The concepts upon which the practice is based, the kind of information that is collected, the nursing needs which are identified, and the nursing care plan for the individual, the family, and the community are different in each situation, but the process remains essentially the same.

The two major responsibilities of the community health nurse are the family and the community; therefore, the process of community health nursing has been presented separately as it relates to the family and to the community. This approach is used purposefully to allow for clarification and depth of exploration. It does not in any way negate the interrelationship between the family and the community, or the fact that in reality community health nurses often work with the family and community simultaneously. Nursing is a unified whole and not a series of separate steps. However, a breakdown of the process helps one to recognize how dependent each step is upon the other, how inseparable the steps are from the nursing action that will result, and how complex each step is in itself. The nature of nursing is derived from the health problems of people, and there is no set of blueprints for action that is universally applicable to each situation. Each family and community must be approached as a separate entity. The nursing actions can come only from a systematic study of the situation—this is the nursing process.

We have made some basic assumptions about the practice of community health nursing which must be kept in mind in all the steps of the nursing process. These assumptions are:

1. The nature of community health nursing practice is derived from the health problems of families and communities.
2. The health of the family as reflected in the health of the community.
3. The family as a whole is different from the individuals whom it comprises.
4. The family has the right and responsibility to make its own decisions.
5. The community health nurse works with the family in determining its nursing needs, in developing the plan of action, and in evaluating the outcomes.
6. Each individual has the right to good health care.
7. Health care should be continuous, comprehensive, and available.
8. The community health nurse works as a member of a health team.

9. The community health nursing program is based upon the needs of the community.
10. There should be a direct relationship between the priority of services provided by the community health nurse and the priority of health problems which have been established by the community.
11. The people in the community are indispensable in all phases of the community health nursing program.

CHAPTER 5

THE FAMILY AS THE PATIENT

The family as the patient of the community health nurse is based upon the concept developed in the early 1920s that the family is the unit of service for the public health nurse. This concept, though laudable and embraced as a basic principle by public health nurses, never became fully operational. One of the reasons was no doubt the prevailing definition of health at that time, which stated that health was the absence of disease. Even though disease was beginning to be understood as having multiple causes, it was not clear how the promotion of health could be conceptualized in relation to providing nursing services to the family as a whole. Another reason may have been that the educational preparation of nurses, including public health nurses, was geared to providing nursing care to the sick individual; thus, the individual was of primary concern. Public health nurses, because their base of operation was in the home, became skillful in recognizing factors in the family that affected the sick individual, and also some of the effects the sick individual had on the family. However, nursing care for the family as a group was difficult to grasp and remained a very elusive concept.

In the highly industrialized and technologic society of today with new knowledge progressing geometrically, the traditional roles of all health workers are changing rapidly. Health is no longer defined as just the absence of disease but also encompasses the physical, social, and emotional well-being of individuals, families, or other groups, and of society at large. Nursing education programs still put undue emphasis on nursing care of sick individuals, but the responsibility of nursing in the prevention of disease and the promotion of health of individuals and of groups is receiving increasing emphasis.

In the following discussion of the family as the patient, we are conceptualizing the family as a small group possessing certain generic characteristics in common with all groups. Thus, the same process is applicable to any group with which the community health nurse is working. Her sphere of competence is her knowledge and ability in working with the total family/group in contrast to working with an individual within a family/group.

When the community health nurse regards the family as a patient, she puts the major focus on the total family and its health problems and nursing needs. The health of families is what will determine the health of communities. The health problems of one member affect his level of functioning, and this influences the functioning of the family as a whole. If the nurse concentrates only on the individual and his needs, she is missing the total picture of the family and may be basing her nursing service on some false assumptions. An analogy can be made to someone buying a house. If he looks at only one room—even though the one room may seem to be the center of activity in the house—and then makes a judgement about the rest of the house, he will be buying or rejecting it on the basis of some false assumptions. In the case of buying a house, the main loss may be only financial. In the case of the family, the main loss may be a lowering of its level of functioning as a unit.

In order for the community health nurse to carry out her responsibilities with the family as a patient, she must have knowledge in areas such as:

1. the life styles of families
2. growth and development of individuals and of families
3. interpersonal relationships
4. groups and how they function
5. the internal and external forces that are always present in any family situation
6. cultural and religious patterns
7. concepts and theories from the behavioral, physical, and biologic sciences basic to nursing practice
8. the environment and its effect on the behavior of human beings
9. the influences of the community on the values, mores, motivation, and health behavior of families
10. medical conditions
11. treatment of disease

Whether the community health nurse is employed in a public health agency, a comprehensive health center, a school, an occupational health setting, a mental health center, an ambulatory service, or a home care program, or works with groups of persons such as drug addicts, expectant parents, or members of communes, her major focus and competence is related to the total family and its relationship to the individual and the community. The nursing process remains constant even though the settings may change.

The definition of a family used throughout this book is one developed by Winch, which states:

> A family is a group of two or more persons, joined by ties of marriage, blood, or adoption, who constitute a single household, who interact with each other in their respective familial roles, and who create and maintain a common culture.[1]

The universal functions of a family as defined by Goode[2] are:

1. reproduction or replacement of members of society
2. status placement
3. biological and emotional maintenance
4. socialization and care of children
5. social control

The major emphasis of the nurse in working with families is on the prevention of disease and the maintenance and promotion of health. She assists the family to maintain and/or increase its health, which in turn will contribute to its ability to carry out its functions. The level at which a family carries out its functions undoubtedly has important implications for its health and well-being. Kaplan and Cassel have presented four studies in which certain elements of family structure and functioning, such as parent-child relationship, fragmentation, life crises, and family competence were found to be related to different aspects of the health status of family members.[3]

The family, as the basic unit in society, shapes and is shaped by all the forces surrounding it. In this interchange the values, beliefs, and customs of society influence the role and functions of the family. At the same time the values, beliefs, and customs held by the family are helping to determine the direction of society. For example, the behavior of people that is sanctioned by society will influence the behavior of members of the family. The tacit sanction by society, for instance, of the communal form of group living has greatly altered the traditional child-rearing functions of the family. The adulation of the young by society has completely altered the function of the family in relation to parents and grandparents. Society with its beliefs, values, and customs invades every aspect of the life of the family, such as the age at which children may go to work, and the age at which they are legally responsible for their own decisions and debts. Society also sanctions what is meant by illness, what an ill person may and may not do, and which treatment he is permitted to receive.

On the other hand, the family is exerting forces equally strong on society, and these forces may influence or change the behaviors sanctioned by society. For example, if families inculcate in their children the value of settling disputes by peaceful means, the pursuit of war by society becomes more difficult. The beliefs and practices of families with regard to the role of women have made dramatic changes in the way society views women today.

It must be kept in mind, however, that the forces operating in society and in the family are constantly intermingling and changing. It often is impossible to determine which exerts the stronger influence, because of the symbiotic relationship between the family and society.

At present there is a great debate going on about the place and role of the family in society, but the larger question seems to be whether the family will survive into the next century. The nontraditional forms of families, such as communes, one-parent families, and the reversal of the traditional roles of the parents, are being singled out by the prophets of doom as the beginning of the end of the family and its universal functions. The available evidence, however, suggests that there is no question about the survival of the family as a social institution. Young[4] argues that the toughness and resilience of the family has few parallels and that man has not discovered any satisfactory substitute. She thinks that the family is probably on the brink of its most important era, particularly in its role of teaching its members the values of the use of abundance for a life worth living.

Cogswell and Sussman[5] also are unqualified in their confidence about the survival of the family. The meaning it will have for its members, the roles and structure, and its durability, however, are uncertain at this time.

Cooper[6] believes that the commune is a sound alternative form to replace the family.

Young[7] takes the opposite view and describes the lack of a unifying principle as the weakness of communes.

The great forces of a modern industrial nation, with its emphasis on individual achievement and freedom of choice, have been effective in shaping and molding family patterns in such a way that what might be called a typical American family—the autonomous nuclear family—has emerged. This nuclear family consists of a mother, a father, and their offspring. Its organization is geared to the needs of a complex, urban, industrialized society. In contrast, the organization of the extended family, which consists of parents, grandparents, children, aunts, uncles, and cousins, is more geared to a rural, agricultural society, which is disappearing rapidly in America.

As a small social unit within the larger society, the functions of the nuclear family have become increasingly specialized. Many of its former functions, such as education of children, occupational opportunities, transportation, provision of goods and services, recreation, care of family members during illness, physical and financial responsibility for aging parents and close relatives, and help in times of crisis, are being taken over by nonfamily organizations. These changes are consistent with the changing society of today. Women, relieved of many household tasks by technologic developments, are freer and better prepared to seek employment outside the home as soon as their children reach school age. Proliferating educational institutions, mass media, and communication systems have assumed increasing responsibility for the development of a common culture and the education of today's children. Children have become more involved in individual pursuits, and spend less and less time under the umbrella of parental guidance and authority. Because of advances in transportation, urbanization, and industrialization, husbands often commute considerable distances to their place of work, and thus are less and less available to assume what was once their traditional role—the head of the household. As a result the basic and vital functions of a family which are necessary for the survival of society, such as sexual satisfaction, procreation, care and socialization of children, and the psychologic and physical security of its members, are now highly specialized functions.

Every relationship within the nuclear family becomes more intensified and continuous without members of an extended family available to cushion some of the impact. There are no relatives available to participate in child rearing and to provide counsel and emotional support to the adult members. The relationships and values within the small specialized social unit, which are so important for emotional security and role socialization, must also be congruent with the relationships and values in the larger society. For example, in America status is earned through individual achievement, with a high premium placed upon individual accomplishment. The nuclear family tends to be organized along these same lines with emphasis on the accomplishments of each individual, rather than on what the family achieves as a group. Thus, a child who receives high grades in school, or who excels in athletics, may have a higher status in the family than the less able members. Within this context it may even be possible for the child to have a higher status than his parents. A continuous rise and fall in status is also possible in this kind of situation.

In addition to the forces in society, there are also forces within the family itself which affect its ability to carry out its functions. For example, patterns of interaction may be changed by the arrival of a new baby, when illness strikes, or when parents get old. As a result the family equilibrium is upset, and new relationships of interaction must be formed. Until the equilibrium is restored it may be difficult or even impossible for the family to carry out its function as a family.

It is of the essence that the community health nurse understand the dynamics of the family and all the forces from within and without that are impinging upon it. She then works with this unit in its wholeness and not merely with its parts. She is the one professional worker who has access to the homes of people in all walks of life and who sees them in all phases of health and illness. She has a long tradition of working with families in their own homes and is accepted by them as a friend and a helping person. At the same time she must be aware of some of the factors which mitigate against her providing services to the family as the patient. These factors must be examined critically, and necessary changes made which will enable the community health nurse to use her competencies to the fullest in helping families move toward a high level of health.

The factors are discussed briefly under the following headings:

1. Results of specialization
2. Effects of agency policies on practice
3. Influence of medical model on nursing
4. Implications of federal legislation
5. Utilization and preparation of community health nurses

RESULTS OF SPECIALIZATION

The health care system today is under attack from all sides, with demands made by the public for more comprehensive services than are readily available. Much of the criticism is being directed at the difficulties clients encounter on entering the health care system, and the fragmentation of services they receive. It is becoming fashionable to point to the medical profession, with its emphasis on specialization, as the culprit in what is commonly referred to as the nonsystem of health care. However, if one looks at the other subsystems which make up the health care system, it becomes evident that specialism is a pervasive theme. Services and personnel have proliferated without any plan for concerted community action. Many specialized professional health workers are appearing on the scene. Each professes that the family is his base of operation; however, how this concept is made operational is unclear. Nonprofessional, indigenous neighborhood workers, who can relate to the people in their own communities, are multiplying daily. They also see the family as their main concern.

Specialization of services and of health workers has resulted in the priorities for services being focused on the functions of a specific agency or the special interest of a particular worker, rather than on the health needs of the family. Thus, clients and patients have many insurmountable hurdles to leap in order to receive the care they need. At the same time, care becomes more fragmented with overlapping, duplication, and gaps in the available health services. Many social agencies, for instance, are geared to provide service to only one segment of the population, for example, to one ethnic or religious group, or to one specific age group. Others may be geared to providing only one service, such as marriage counseling, or adoption and placement of children. Similarly, health agencies that have a special interest in one disease category or age group concentrate their energies and personnel in that direction.

The nursing care system also reflects the proliferation and specialization of nurses and nursing services in a community. With a few exceptions, nursing has not taken the initiative for both short- and long-range planning for nursing services that will meet the nursing needs of the people in the community. In fact, the opposite is the usual pattern. The late Congressman John Fogarty stated that there was no community in the United States that could say with pride that all its nursing needs were being met adequately. The same statement could be accurately made today.

With increasing specialization in nursing, more and more nurses have the community as their arena. They are engaged in various kinds of programs set up to meet the needs of such special groups of people as mothers and infants, poverty groups, senior citizens, and special disease categories. With no overall community planning the nursing services to families become further fragmented with several nurses, as well as other health workers, visiting the family for one specific function. Thus, there is much duplication of effort, overlapping, and wide gaps in the types of nursing services available to the people. The concomitant results are waste of precious, scarce nurse power, prohibitive costs, lack of job satisfaction, large turnover of personnel, and an unclear definition of what nursing has to offer.

EFFECTS OF AGENCY POLICIES ON PRACTICE

Policies are necessary to give direction to the community health nursing program. The policies must be consistent with the purposes of the agency and must also make it possible for the nurse to provide nursing service to the family as a whole. Because policies directly influence the type and quality of nursing services rendered to families, they must be evaluated frequently to assure that the best interests of the people and community are their primary focus. Staff nurses and consumers, as well as administrators, should be included in the evaluation and revision of existing policies and the development of new ones.

Policies that make it difficult for the community health nurse to give service to the entire family relate to such things as: the number of visits that can be made to a particular family; the priorities of the agency program; the category or age group of patients that can be admitted to the case load; the kind of nursing service that can be provided; the length of time a patient may be on the active case load; the working hours of the agency; the kinds of records that are kept; the fee system; the types of decisions that must be made only by the supervisor; and the policies relating to who can render what kind of service.

In looking at policies one must also keep in mind that long-standing practices sometimes have the force of policy and may affect the kind of nursing care the nurse renders. Some of these, such as the length of a visit, accompanying a patient to the clinic, making appointments for patients and families, procedures in the home, and the method of recording visits, have a direct influence on the service the family receives from the community health nurse. Other practices have a more indirect influence by affecting the professional development of the nurse and thus affecting the service she gives. Examples are the practices which dictate who participates in neighborhood or community meetings, who participates in teaching of groups, how in-service education programs are planned and carried out, the amount of time allowable for pursuit of academic courses, or attendance at professional meetings, and the role of the supervisor in making decisions about services the individual nurse should render to her families.

A growing number of community health nurses, particularly the recent graduates, are becoming more vocal about the health problems and nursing needs of families and communities. They are making unprecedented demands that they be given the resources to meet the total nursing needs of the families they serve. The people themselves are also clamoring for more comprehensive and less fragmented services. Community health nursing must join, and sometimes lead, the growing parade of "risk takers," and change its policies so that its practitioners can use their education and experience in creative practices which are relevant to the needs of people in society today.

INFLUENCE OF THE MEDICAL MODEL ON NURSING

Nursing practice has been defined largely by two aspects of medicine. One is the major emphasis on the diagnosis and treatment of disease in the individual; the other is the unequivocal fact that only the physician can make the diagnosis and prescribe the treatment. This is the model upon which the whole system of health care is organized. With this model as a guide, the education of nurses has been geared to preparing them to work with individuals who are sick and under the care of a physician.

With its reliance on the individual, the medical model mitigates against the community health nurse providing total nursing service to the entire family as a group. The illness of the individual and the treatment of his disease receive first priority. All the information about the individual is given to the physician, who in turn makes the decisions about what the individual's treatment shall be and what he shall be told about his illness. The right of the individual or the family to have all the information and then to make its own decisions is not part of this model.

The concept of autonomous functions and responsibilities of the community health nurse in relation to prevention of disease and promotion of health does not coincide with the medical model and can be a source of conflict. This conflict is apparent in the generally accepted policies which state that the nurse may visit only patients who are under the care of a physician. "Keeping the well person well," a key concept of community health nursing, is not possible in this context.

The community health nurse can no longer base her practices on the medical model, but must accept the responsibility and accountability for making nursing judgments in relation to the health needs of families. She may do this in collaboration with other professional and nonprofessional workers, including the physician. Her nursing care plan will reflect her role as provider of nursing care and health teacher, as well as coordinator of the services provided by other members of the nursing and health team.

IMPLICATIONS OF FEDERAL LEGISLATION

As discussed in the preceding chapters, the role of the federal government and its effect in all areas of the life of the people has undergone a dramatic shift from the "hands-off" policy in the last century to the strong central government of today. There are indications of the fact that the values inherent in rugged individualism have not lost their glitter; but there is little room for questioning the paramount responsibility of the federal government in promoting the general welfare of all the people. However, the debates about how the government should carry out its responsibility are opinionated, controversial, and charged with emotion.

The American people are in general agreement that health is a right of all people, but as yet there is no health policy for the nation as a whole. Consequently, categorical federal legislation and funding for specific age groups (such as Medicare, Medicaid, or Children and Youth) or for specific diseases (such as heart disease, cancer, and stroke) are contributing to the duplication, overlapping, and gaps in services and the specialism of professional workers.

Federal legislation, health insurance plans, and third-party payments, with all their restrictions and limitations, are tending to restrict the services of the community health nurse to one age group or one disease category. How to meet the health problems and nursing needs of people who do not happen to fall into the categories for which funds are available is a problem of growing concern. One of the earliest principles of public health nursing was that the services of the public health nurse should be available to everyone in the community. The application of this principle always varied from community to community, but it was an essential part of all organized public health nursing services.

Community health nursing must constantly keep this principle in mind and take steps to assure that the availability of money does not determine the priorities for service. It is obvious that if all the energies of the community health nurse are used in taking care of the sick person who is bedridden, or concentrated on one specific group, then her services will not contribute to the improvement of the health of all the people in the community. In spite of the many pressures that result from categorical federal legislation and from the demands of special interest groups, it is imperative that health priorities be established that will contribute to keeping well people well and not just to the curing of disease.

PREPARATION AND UTILIZATION OF COMMUNITY HEALTH NURSES

At the present time the health manpower needs of society are undergoing critical scrutiny, and from all groups we are hearing about the scarcity of adequate numbers of health professionals. The utilization and distribution of manpower are also getting increased attention.

Nursing is the only profession that requires its practitioners to have theory and practice in community health as part of their generic preparation. In 1972, there were 50,986 nurses employed full time in public health.[8] This is an increase of 7,227 over 1968. The largest increase—4,505—was in nurses employed by local boards of education. Of the total number, 50,986, 47,302 were employed in local agencies. The largest number, 19,355, were employed by boards of education; 19,277 were employed by local health departments, and 4,247 by nonofficial agencies. The remainder were employed in either an organized categorical program, an organized home care program, or a combination agency.

The national ratio was 23.2 full-time public health nurses per 100,000 population. Twenty-one states had higher ratios than the national average.

As mentioned previously, the employing agency and its policies and purposes exert a great deal of influence on the practices of the community health nurse and her ability to provide service to the family as the patient. For example, boards of education, with approximately 19,355 nurses, concentrate their energies on the school-age segment of the population. In most instances, it is difficult or impossible for the nurse to have contact with any member of the family other than the child. She may know the strengths and weaknesses of the total family of a few of the children, and have some ideas about a few others. With few exceptions, however, the majority of her activities are confined to the child in the school.

The remaining 38,986 nurses on the local level are employed either by an official, a voluntary, or a combination agency, or by a hospital-based home care program. Each subscribes in some degree to the family as the patient and exerts its energies toward that end. In actuality, however, priorities for services may be established on the basis of sources of funding, legislation, or special interest groups. The educational preparation of the staff nurses also makes it more difficult to embrace the family as the patient.

In spite of these obstacles, community health nurses represent the best single source for providing leadership in meeting community health problems. By establishing a milieu in which community health nurses are encouraged to critically assess their practices and to take advantage of every opportunity to exert the leadership for which their education and experience has prepared them, many of these obstacles can be overcome. A reordering of priorities, and the development of administrative structures which permit the utmost utilization of the competencies of each nurse in community health are the first steps that must be taken. In this era of scarcity of manpower and of urgent need to utilize fully the competencies of each worker, all professionals are reassessing their roles and responsibilities. A better-educated, more sophisticated population with rising expectations is demanding changes in the health care system. Maximum feasible participation is becoming the watchword for many consumer groups. Accountability of professional practice is gaining momentum, with people no longer willing to accept mediocre or inappropriate services. The focus of health care is beginning to move toward the needs of the patient and client as the primary goal; and away from the primacy of the needs of the professional and the agency or institution which employs them.

SUMMARY

Community health nursing in the early 1920s was in the vanguard in broadening the nation's concept of health. It has the potential for the same kind of leadership today, with the largest group of professional workers who have educational preparation in the theory and practice of community health and community health nursing. It has access to people from all walks of life in their own homes, and first-hand knowledge of the health needs of people and of the communities in which they live. It has a long tradition of working with families and collaborating with citizen groups and other professionals. Unlike some of the other health workers in this period of turmoil and change, the community health nurse is still held in high regard by the community and its people. In the words of one militant community leader: "community health nurses still have a chance."

If the emphasis of the community health nurse is to be on the family as a whole, with the prevention of disease and the promotion and maintenance of health as the first priority, there are some changes in practices (which do not require a large outlay of money) that she must institute immediately. She must: give high priority to the independent functions of nursing and pursue them aggressively; become the advocate for the family in all health matters and keep the total family as the main goal; participate with others in planning community health programs; take leadership in interpreting nursing and defining nursing needs; become involved with consumer groups in the community who are concerned with health; seek opportunities to exert leadership in areas where nursing can make a contribution; publicize the factors in the community which contribute to poor health; get acquainted with legislators and support good health legislation; become actively involved in the legislative process: experiment with new ways of delivering health and nursing services to families; and develop friendships with the persons responsible for the press and other mass media.

REFERENCES

1. R. F. Winch, *The Modern Family* (New York: Henry Holt and Company, 1952), p. 14.
2. W. J. Goode, "The Sociology of the Family—Horizons in Family Theory," In Merton, R. K., *et al. Sociology Today: Problems and Prospects* (New York: Harper and Row, 1965), Ch. 7 pp. 188–89.
3. B. H. Kaplan and J. C. Cassel, (eds.), *Family and Health: An Epidemiological Approach* (Chapel Hill: Institute for Research in Social Science, University of North Carolina, 1975).

4. L. Young, *The Fractured Family* (New York: McGraw-Hill Book Company, 1973), pp. 137–38.
5. B. E. Cogswell and M. B. Sussman, "Changing Family and Marriage Forms: Complications for Human Service Systems," In M. B. Sussman, (ed), *Non-traditional Family Forms in the 1970's* (Minneapolis: National Council on Family Relations, 1972), p. 137.
6. D. Cooper, *The Death of the Family* (New York: Vintage Books, 1971), pp. 44–45.
7. Young, op. cit., p. 148.
8. American Nurses' Association, *ANA Facts About Nursing 1974–75* (Kansas City, Mo.: American Nurses' Association, 1976).

BIBLIOGRAPHY

Ackerman, N. *The Psychodynamics of Family Life.* New York: Basic Books, 1958.

Aldous, J. *The Developmental Approach to Family Analysis.* Athens, Ga: Department of Child Development, University of Georgia, 1975 (mimeo).

American Nurses' Association. *Facts About Nursing 1974–75.* Kansas City, Mo.: American Nurses' Association, 1976.

Blisten, D. R. *The World of the Family.* New York: Random House, 1963.

Cavan, R. R. *The American Family.* New York: Thomas Y. Crowell Company, 1955.

Chapman, J., and Chapman, H. St. Louis: C. V. Mosby Company, 1975.

Cogswell, B. E., and Sussman, M. B. "Changing Family and Marriage Forms: Complications for Human Service Systems," In M. B. Sussman, ed. *Non-Traditional Family Forms in the 1970's.* Minneapolis: National Council on Family Relations, 1972.

Cohn, H., and Schmidt, W. M. "The Practice of Family Health Care—A Descriptive Study. *Amer. J. Public Health* 65 (April 1975):375–83.

Cooper, D. *The Death of the Family.* New York: Vintage Books, 1971.

Coser, R. L. *The Family: Its Structure and Function.* New York: St. Martin's Press, 1964.

Duvall, E. M. *Family Development.* 4th ed. Philadelphia: J. B. Lippincott Company, 1972.

Goode W. J. "The Sociology of the Family—Horizons in Family Theory." In Merton, R. K., *et al., Sociology Today: Problems and Prospects.* New York: Harper & Row, 1965. Ch. 7, pp. 178–96.

Hymovich, D. P., and Barnard, M., eds. *Family Health Care.* New York: McGraw-Hill Book Company, 1973.

Kaplan, B. H., and Cassel, J. C., eds. *Family and Health: An Epidemiological Approach.* Chapel Hill: Institute for Research in Social Science, University of North Carolina, 1975.

Kirkpatric, C. *The Family as Process and Institution.* New York: The Ronald Press, 1967.

Laing, R. D. *The Politics of the Family and Other Essays*. New York: Vintage Books, 1972.

LeMasters, E. E. *Parents in Modern America*. Homewood, Ill.: The Dorsey Press, 1974. Chap. 4.

Matthis, E. "The Problem Oriented System in Public Health Nursing." In *The Problem-Oriented System—a Multidisciplinary Approach*. New York: National League for Nursing,1974. Pp. 48–54.

Murata, J. E. "The Nurse as Family Practitioner." *Amer. J. Nurs.* 74 (February 1974):254–57.

Nathanson, E. "Getting a Bill through Congress." *Amer. J. Nurs.* 75 (July 1975):1109–11.

Nye, F. I., and Berardo, F. M. *Emerging Conceptual Frameworks in Family Analysis*. New York: The Macmillan Company, 1966.

Pittman, R. "The Man in the Family." *Nursing Outlook,* 16 (April 1968): 62–64.

Pratt, L. "Conjugal Organization and Health." *J. Marriage & the Family* 34 (January 1972):85:–94.

Reinhardt, A. M. and Quinn, M. D. *Family-Centered Community Nursing: A Sociological Framework.* St. Louis: C. V. Mosby, 1973.

Robischon, P. "Community Nursing in a Changing Climate." *Nursing Outlook* 19 (June 1971):410–13.

Roy, R., and Rustum, D. "Is Monogamy Outdated?" In Schultz, D. A., and Wilson, R. D., eds. *Readings on the Changing Family*. Englewood Cliffs, N.J.: Prentice-Hall, 1975. Pp. 300–13.

Ruano, B. J. "This I Believe . . . about Nurses Innovating Change." *Nursing Outlook* 19 (June 1971):416–18.

Winch, R. F. *The Modern Family*. New York: Henry Holt and Company, 1952.

Young, L. *The Fractured Family*. New York: McGraw-Hill Book Company, 1973.

CHAPTER 6

FAMILY DATA COLLECTION

In nursing, in contrast to such professions as law and medicine, there is no general consensus about the kind of information nurses need to have about their patients in order to carry out their professional nursing responsibilities. The base line of information needed by each physician about his patient and by each lawyer about his client has been generally agreed upon by their respective professions. The skill in analyzing and interpreting the data varies from one lawyer to another and from one physician to another, but the base-line information each profession has agreed upon remains fairly constant.

The writers, as a result of their experience as community health nursing practitioners and educators, believe a similar data base of information is necessary for the community health nurse to provide comprehensive care to her families.[1] Otherwise, each nurse will collect only the information which she thinks is important. The skill in the analysis and interpretation of the data base will vary from one nurse to another, and is dependent upon her knowledge, judgment, and experience.

The collection and analysis of the data-base about a family helps the community health nurse to assess and diagnose the family's health problems and nursing needs in a systematic, organized fashion based upn a solid foundation of knowledge. A plan of action can then be made which takes into consideration the individual strengths and weaknesses of each family and its ability to cope with its problems. The data-base may be obtained from direct questioning, through observation, by discussion with relatives, and significant others, from hospital and other health care records, from other health professionals, and so forth.

The information the community health nurse should know about a family can be categorized under four headings:

1. Family characteristics.
2. Socioeconomic and cultural factors.
3. Environmental factors.
4. Medical and health history.

It is essential for the nurse to have the information under these categories for each of her families. The analysis of the data may point up areas where further information is needed, but each item under the categories will give some clues about a family. However, it must be kept in mind that the importance of the data in determining health problems and nursing needs lies in the relationship of one item or category to another. The community health nurse cannot determine this relationship until she has all the information.

In developing the items, we have kept in mind that with many families the nurse has only one contact while with others she may have regular contacts over a long period of time. Community health nurses have always made decisions about whether families have a nursing need and about the number of visits necessary to alleviate the need. However, they often remark that they cannot get information on one visit (although, in many instances, after one contact a decision is made that no further visits are necessary). Collection of data in a systematic way will help to highlight the information the nurse requires in order to make a sound professional judgment about nursing needs. We have also kept in mind the dynamic nature of the family, and recognize that the community health nurse who has continuing contact with a family will have increased knowledge and understanding of its problems and way of life.

In gathering data about a family, the nurse must keep in mind that no two families are alike. On the other hand, according to Duvall,[2] there is a predictability about family development that helps one to know what to expect of any family at a given stage in its development. Each family goes through each stage in its own way, but each follows a universal sequence of family development. This is true irrespective of where a family is found—in an inner-city ghetto, in a rural farm, in a suburb, whether in the North, South, East, or West. There are many internal and external forces operating in a family at any one time that produce a dynamic, changing situation to which the community health nurse must be constantly alert.

The data-base information about a family which we believe is essential for each community health nurse to have in order to define its health problems and nursing needs may be similar to the information that a social worker, a nutritionist, or other professional worker would collect. In fact, there are many complaints from patients and clients that they have to repeat the same information every time they meet a different worker or go to a new agency or institution. Each professional discipline, however, has a different purpose for collecting the data and, thus, asks different questions about it. In other words, the uniqueness of each discipline lies in the pertinent questions it asks about similar data.

In the following pages the items under each category are discussed, and some of the important clues in regard to health status are pointed out. Following the discussion of each item are some pertinent questions the community health nurse might ask in her assessment of the information she has collected.

FAMILY CHARACTERISTICS

Demographic data such as age, sex, marital status, and position in the family of each member are fairly easy to obtain. This information presents a composite picture of the members of the household and gives some clues about the developmental stage of the family. For example, if the demographic data show that the family consists of the parents and two preschool children, we know that they are at a different developmental stage and will have needs different from those of a family unit of a husband and wife whose children have married and started families of their own. These data also provide information about who lives in the household, and the relationship of each person to the head of the household. Duvall[3] has stated that information about who lives in the family home is one of the three things that will predict what is going on in a family. The two others are where a family is in time, i.e., its life cycle within an era of social change and in a given season, day, and hour; and how a family rates in the community as indicated by its social status.

Each person has specific needs in relation to his age and sex. How these needs are met within the family are harbingers to its health problems. The infant, whose needs can be met only by others, requires more constant attention than the teen-ager, who can satisfy some of his needs by participation in peer-group activities. An aged parent who is a member of the household can be either a positive or negative force in the movement of the family toward a high level of well-being. The size of a family may have some bearing on its health. For example, small families have fewer health problems and tend to seek care from a physician more often than large families.

The work history should be obtained for each adult member in the household to assess the potential influence of the hazards of the occupation or work environment on the health of the worker and/or his family. The type of work should be clearly determined, and such descriptions as "retired," "engineer," "teacher," and so forth should be avoided. The work history of a retired individual, for example, will give clues about his possible exposure to chemicals or other hazardous substances. The same thing applies to engineer, teacher, and all other occupations.

The demographic data give some background information about the family that is necessary before any analysis can be done. Armed with this information, the community health nurse can then ask pertinent questions about the other data in this category.

The roles and relationships of family members are less easy to obtain and may depend upon skillful observation and astute questioning by the nurse. One of the functions of the family is the preparation of the next generation for its role in society. The values of the community are inherent guidelines that the family uses in role assignment. The roles and relationships must be congruent with those of society if the family is to fulfill its function. Each member has a different role according to his age group and place in the family. The roles are not static, however, and at any one time while a member is functioning in one role he may also be undergoing a role transition from one age group to another. The community health nurse, because of her access to families in all walks of life and in all stages of sickness and health, has an opportunity to observe the members in their assigned roles and to assess the ability of the individual to assume his role. In some families the roles are clearly understood by the members, and there is an orderly role transition from one age group to another. Where roles are not clear there is apt to be role diffusion with overlapping and conflict. The parents serve an important function as the adult role models for their children. In families with only one parent the role of the other parent is either abandoned or performed by some other person. In some families there is a close relative who takes the place of the missing parent. In other instances there is a member of the household who is not a family member but who plays a significant role in the stability of the family, perhaps replacing the missing parent as a role model. It is not uncommon for one of the older children to abandon his role as a teen-ager and assume the role of father or mother.

Roles and relationships that are clearly defined in the day-by-day functioning of the family may be disrupted when a crisis occurs, such as the arrival of a new baby, illness in the family, or the death of a member. How the family manages when faced with a crisis situation gives some concrete evidence about its health problems and coping ability.

Questions the community health nurse might ask about this information include the following: Are the roles of each individual clearly defined, or is there overlapping? Are the roles appropriate for each age? What role models do the parents project? How do the family members get along with each other? Is there a feeling of family unity or does each individual go his own way? How do members communicate with each other? What is the relationship of the parent to the children? Is one member made the scapegoat for all the family problems?

In her assessment of a family the community health nurse must take into consideration who makes what kinds of decisions and how these are made about the family. Herein may lie the key to the total health picture. The decisions a family makes about the individual member or about the family as a whole are intimately associated with its life style. By and large the nurse has her most frequent contact with the mother. If the father is the one who makes all the decisions in the family, ways must be evolved for the nurse to have contact with the father. On the other hand, if decisions are a "family affair," this may increase or decrease her effectiveness.

Very few studies have been done in relation to how decisions are made in a family. In some that have been done in middle-class families, it has been found that in the first years of marriage the husband and wife jointly make the decisions. At about the time the second child is born, joint decision making is on the wane, with each parent having fairly clearly defined areas in which they reign more or less supreme. However, major decisions will still be made jointly.

The literature is replete with stories and stereotypes about persons who make the decisions in a family. In many situations the father is cast as the authoritarian decision maker who rules with an iron hand and of whom everyone is in awe. There are other situations in which the mother is depicted as the decision maker. She is as authoritarian as the father but her methods are more subtle, so she is much beloved. In still fewer instances the family as a whole is a council or committee that has responsibility for all family decisions.

In the nuclear family of today, with its emphasis on the individual and his achievements, these stereotypes do not have much relevance, although we still find vestiges of them. Instead, decisions are often made by the individual on the basis of his own needs rather than on the needs of the family as a whole.

Questions the nurse might ask regarding decision making are: How are decisions made in the family? Does the responsibility for decisions rest with an appropriate person or persons? How does the pattern of decision making affect the family as a whole?

As with everything else, the daily activities of a family will vary tremendously, but each family has a pattern of sleeping, of eating, and of use of leisure time. Rest and sufficient sleep are requirements for each individual. Successful nursing intervention is related to a knowledge of the sleeping patterns of a family. The information gathered about the sleeping patterns gives the community health nurse clues about the amount of rest each member has and how his sleep pattern is related to that of the total family. If one member sleeps poorly, the effect of this on the total family should be assessed. For example, if an infant needs constant attention at night, this could result in loss of sleep by the father. He would then be more prone to accidents at his place of work the next day. Carried to its logical conclusion, his lack of sleep could have an effect on the economy of the community.

Questions about this item might be: Are the sleeping arrangements appropriate for each age group? Does anyone have a nap during the day? Are there regular hours for retiring and getting up in the morning, or is this dependent upon the desires and whims of the individual? Is age a factor in determining the time of going to bed? If family members sleep together, what effect does this have on them and on the rest of the family?

Closely allied to the sleeping pattern is the eating pattern. If each person arises at a different time in the morning, this will affect the time he has his first meal. Similarly, the last food he has in the evening may be related to the time he retires. In some sections of the country it is customary to have a siesta as part of a prolonged lunch period. This may affect both the time of retiring and the time when the next meal is consumed.

The dietary patterns and food habits of families are closely allied to their total life style. Taboos and restrictions about food, which may have no relation to its nutritive value, are passed on from one generation to the next. Ethnic background and religious beliefs exert a great deal of influence on what families eat, and how and when it is eaten. Food has many different meanings for people and is often tied up with family celebrations and special holidays. Children learn very early in life that they can win approval or disapproval from parents by the amount of food they consume. Many times food is the reward an individual receives for behavior that is sanctioned by the family. On the other hand, withholding food is used as a punishment, such as going to bed without any supper. One of the reasons it is so difficult for some persons who are overweight to restrict their food intake in order to lose weight is because they have a deeply ingrained belief that they are being punished when food is restricted or withheld.

From her observations of the family eating habits, of the kitchen area, and comments made by the mother, the community health nurse can get some ideas about the food habits. An analysis of the food eaten over a 24-hour period will give valuable information about the nutritive value of the food eaten by the family. Observations of the family members help identify those who are obese and those who are underweight.

Questions of concern to the nurse might be: Does each member, and the family as a whole, have sufficient and nutritious food? How many meals does the family have each day? Which is the heartiest? Does the family sit down at the table together at mealtime? Who is overweight? Who is underweight?

With advancing technology and the shorter work week, more people have increasing amounts of leisure time, and there is every indication that this trend will continue. How the family spends its leisure time may help the nurse know how best to plan for any health teaching that might be indicated. It also might give her some clues about family unity and the use of community resources. The data about the use of leisure may show that some of the members have too much leisure, while others do not have enough. This may be due to differences in age and sex, or because of long working hours. The roles of each member also affect the amount of leisure time. The way household tasks are assigned may discriminate against some of the individuals. How leisure time is used can give clues about the individual as a person.

Questions regarding leisure time might revolve around the following: Is the use of leisure time appropriate for the sex and age group of the individual? How much time is devoted to watching television? Does any family member have an all-consuming hobby, and what effect does this have on the family? Does the family have any joint activities for leisure time?

SOCIOECONOMIC AND CULTURAL FACTORS

The information about family income and expenses gives some immediate evidence about the adequacy of the income to meet the daily living expenses. The sources of income are a determinant of the likelihood of extra funds being available to meet a financial crisis. The income also indicates the degree of financial responsibility that is assumed by working members other than the head of the household.

The occupation, education, and income of the head of the household help to define the socioeconomic status and give some idea about the placement of the family in the community, its aspirations, and possibilities for social mobility.

The educational level of the parents is a fairly good predictor about the amount of health knowledge they have, and the probability of their actively seeking further information. Persons with a high school education and above tend to read more and to have more health knowledge than those who have less than a high school education.

The income also offers some suggestions about health problems. There is a direct relationship between illness and the level of income, with families in the lower socioeconomic level having more illnesses than those in the upper income brackets. Those with lower incomes also spend a larger percentage of their income on illness.

Knowledge about who has responsibility for planning how the income is spent, and about any outstanding debts of the family, will help the community health nurse in planning with the family ways to alleviate their health problems. How people spend their money is a personal matter that is related to many facets of the total life of the individual. For example, if a family has a future orientation, it will be more apt to put aside some money to meet emergencies that might arise in the future. In contrast, the family that is present-oriented will be more inclined to use its money for gratification of a present need and not be too concerned about the future. Knowledge about the income of a family and how it spends its money is indispensable for the community health nurse if she is to plan with them about alleviating their health problems.

Questions about income are: What does the amount of income tell about this family? Is it adequate? Do they have any financial assets that are available in an emergency? How much does each of the working members contribute, and is his contribution appropriate? What are the working hours of the mother and father? What is the relationship between income and expense? Is impulse buying or "buy now and pay later" a way of life? Does the appropriate person make decisions about the money, and how it is spent? What effect do the outstanding debts have on the amount of money available?

Knowledge about ethnic groups and their culture has always been part of the armamentarium of the community health nurse, and it is assuming more importance at the present time. One of the characteristics of society today is the search by the individual for an identity and his constant query, "Who am I?" This is reflected in the increasing emphasis on being part of an ethnic group, and pride in the cultural heritage associated with that group. Individuals who a few years ago were exerting all their efforts to become assimilated into the mainstream of American life are now embracing their ethnic origins and way of life. The extent to which the ethnic background influences the individual and the family as a whole must be known and understood by the community health nurse in order for her to assess the strengths and weaknesses in the family's ability to cope with its health problems.

Questions she might ask would be: What does the ethnic group heritage mean in this family? Are all its activities governed by ethnic identification? Do they identify with the ethnic group for only specific activities, or do they completely reject this group?

Religion, which at one time was a pervasive force in each person's life, is now the object of much soul searching and questioning. Modes of life that formerly adhered to religious convictions are being abandoned, while at the same time the search for individual identity widens. However, it must be kept in mind that the religious background of an individual or of a family still exerts a powerful influence on behavior. Individuals who have abandoned their religious convictions may still have some guilt feelings because of an early indoctrination to their religious heritage. The community health nurse must be constantly alert to the fact that knowledge about the ethnic and religious background of a family gives valuable clues, but cannot be looked at in a vacuum. She must avoid attaching stereotypes and making generalizations on the basis of limited or incomplete information.

The questions she asks about the information she has collected will help to clarify what religion means to a particular family. What influence does the religious affiliation have on the behavior of the family? What does religion mean to this family? How is it related to the ethnic background? Do all members conform in the same way? How do they explain the differences between their behavior and their religious teachings? If the parents have different religious backgrounds, how is this affecting the family?

Probably the most important determinant of how people behave is related to their value system and what they believe is important and unimportant. For example, if one believes in education, he makes sure his sons and daughters have an education; if he believes prevention of disease is important, he will get his children immunized; and if he believes that owning his own home is important, he will strive toward that goal. It is not possible for the community health nurse to have an understanding of the value system of a family on one contact. However, she can get some clues from the comments of the mother, her observations of the furniture in the home, its condition, the housecleaning, the kind of clothing worn by each member, the make of the automobile they own, the state of repairs inside and outside the home, and the type of neighborhood in which the family lives. The values of a family are closely associated with its life style and aspirations.

The community health nurse has her own hierarchies of values that have a similar influence on her way of thinking and behaving. In order for any nursing intervention to be effective, she must maintain a constant vigil to avoid making judgments about the family based on what she believes is right and wrong. However, having knowledge and understanding about the value system of a family, assessing its strengths and weaknesses in relation to its values, and working with the family within this system does not mean that the community health nurse has to abandon her own values and embrace those of the family with whom she is working. Her professional responsibility is to help families recognize their health problems, and to provide the necessary information and assistance that will enable them to make sound decisions about the alleviation or solution of these problems.

Examples of questions she might ask about the information are: What is the relation of the value system to the ethnic background and religion of the family? How are discrepancies handled? What seem to be the positive values? What about the negative ones?

The family is only one of the many institutions and resources within a community. The autonomous nuclear family, with its limited contact and responsibility for extended family members, is dependent upon extrafamilial agencies, institutions, and social contacts in order to maintain itself. Significant others, such as close friends and neighbors, become important extensions of the family and lend help and assistance in time of need. The relationship of each family to the larger community gives some indication of its place in society as a whole and of the extrafamilial resources that are utilized. Some families have only superficial and limited contact with programs or institutions in the community, and tend to be alienated from anything other than the immediate family and its problems. Others become so completely involved in community activities that home becomes just a place to sleep and to have an occasional meal; while still others seem to have the ability to enrich the quality of life of the family as a unit by the judicious use of community agencies and participation in their activities. Knowledge of the extent of societal contacts helps the community health nurse in her assessment of the strengths and weaknesses of the family's ability to cope with its health problems.

She may ask herself these questions: What does the participation of the family in the community agencies tell one about this family? Is it tied in with their ethnic heritage and religious background? Are there significant others, and what effect do they have on the family? Do all members participate in some community activity? Is it appropriate for each member's age and sex?

ENVIRONMENTAL FACTORS

Shelter is one of the basic needs of all people, and the type and kind of housing play an important part in the life of the family. Housing also affects health, as there is a direct relationship between the kind of housing and the health problems of a family. This is particularly evident in the incidence of illness and disability in children, with a much higher incidence found in those living under poor housing conditions.

The observations of the community health nurse about the living space, the sleeping arrangements, the adequacy of the furniture, the type of refrigeration, the toilet facilities, the presence or absence of flies and rodents, the water supply, and the internal and external accident hazards give valuable insight into what some of the health problems may be and how the family copes with them.

In the assessment of the environmental factors, the information about the type and quality of housing should be looked at in relation to the effect on the particular family. Are the living space, furniture, refrigeration, and toilet facilities adequate? Are the accident hazards due to improper care of the house by the landlord, or are they due to misuse of the property by the family? Does the condition of the dwelling conform to the housing regulations in the community? What clues to possible health problems are available?

The neighborhood and community in which a family lives exert a tremendous influence on the family. In turn, the family is the bridge to the organizations and activities in the community. The influence of the community is seen in the type of dwellings and how they are kept up; the use of health and related facilities; the buying patterns of the people; the feelings about the schools; the incidence of crime; and the way the people view the police and other protective services, to name a few.

Health facilities, social and welfare agencies, recreation areas, and churches may be available in the community, but they may not be utilized by the family because public transportation is inconvenient or inaccessible. Transportation, which has played so important a part in the development of the country since 1865, is still making tremendous strides in transporting people from one section of the world to another. However, an impasse seems to have been reached in public transportation systems in the urban and suburban areas, with less service available each year.

How people feel about using the available community facilities has a great deal to do with their experiences in using neighborhood agencies or institutions. If the experiences have been positive, the use will be greater than if they were dissatisfied with their previous encounters. These feelings may have no relationship to the quality of the program and services offered by the agency or institution.

The total environment of the individual and family, which is receiving increased emphasis today, cannot be ignored in assessing the health problems and nursing needs of families. One cannot identify and treat the health problems of a family without understanding its environment and the effect on the individual and family. The "community of solution" for the majority of health problems of families probably lies in their own neighborhood and the milieu from which the problems developed and were nurtured.

Assessment of the environmental information would include some of the following questions: In what kind of neighborhood does the family live? How do the type and the condition of the housing of the family compare with other dwellings in the neighborhood? Is there pressure from the neighborhood for all families to conform to one standard? If health and social facilities are available, are they used? If public transportation is not available, what other means are used to transport the people?

HEALTH AND MEDICAL HISTORY

The standards of health in a family come from its own background, history, and tradition. Health practices vary from family to family, but there are some common characteristics. Life styles of families and of individuals within the family exert a strong influence on the day-to-day activities which may either enhance or diminish the present and potential health problems. Smoking and overeating are examples of day-to-day practices which may be detrimental to health.

The knowledge a family has about health and the value it puts upon it are important determinants for its health behavior. The level at which a family carries out its functions may also be a clue to the health status of its members. Health is an abstract term that has many different meanings. Everyone is for it, but a clear-cut definition eludes them. By and large, if health is thought of at all, it is related to the absence of disease. Also, each person is apt to define health in relation to his ability to perform in his usual manner. He may have a health problem or health problems as defined by a professional, but by his own definition he is "healthy."

It is necessary for the nurse to understand the meaning of health to a family in order to determine what it perceives to be its health problems. Perhaps it will be necessary to broaden the family's definition of health before any nursing intervention can be implemented.

Questions that will help in evaluating the information are: What is the relationship of the health practices of the family to its knowledge and attitude about health? How accurate is its definition of its health problems?

The medical history of each family member should be obtained in order to have information about the past and present significant illnesses for which medical care was sought. The current illnesses and any treatment and medications being taken should be ascertained. The presence of acute or chronic disease in one member of a family can change the balance of the many forces that are operating at any one time and can cause temporary or permanent disruption in the family.

Some idea about what the family thinks about disease prevention can be arrived at by the immunization status of each individual. When and why a member visits the physician adds to the clues about the value placed on prevention of disease. A physical assessment of family members may be necessary to determine the present health status of the family. The armentarium of the community health nurse should include knowledge and skill in physical assessment, as well as in taking a complete health history. This information will provide a broad data base which will contribute to making sounder nursing judgments about the health problems and nursing needs of the family. "Triage in the home" is an unexplored area. However, the primary care responsibility of the community health nurse opens up new vistas in which her potential contribution in relation to family health is largely unexplored.

The nurse in assessing this information might ask: What is the present state of illness in each member? What relation does the treatment and medication he is receiving have to his present illness? Is the immunization status of each person up to date? What health problems need further exploration? Which family members should see a physician immediately?

Families today are victims of a maze of health care services and facilities. The specialism in medicine makes it virtually impossible to obtain a family physician, and patients are shuttled back and forth from one specialist to another. One of the ironies of this affluent country in the latter third of the twentieth century is that hospital emergency rooms are replacing the family physician. The high cost of medical and dental care is also one of the deterrents to seeking help. The method of paying for medical care is an important factor to be kept in mind in assessing family health needs.

Questions related to medical care might include: What is the source of medical care for the family? Is it different for each individual? What effect does the cost of medical care have on the utilization of physicians' services? Does the health insurance, if any, include the entire family? Are preventive services included?

How the family manages and where and to whom it turns for help in time of illness or crisis must be included in the data base. Relatives or adult family members may be the resource that is used. In some situations neighbors and close friends are the source of help. It is being recognized more and more today that there are specific persons outside the immediate family constellation who exert a considerable influence on the behavior of the individual members and on the family as a whole.

These persons are referred to as "significant others." Speck and Attneave[4] further elaborate on this matter in their discussion of a social network for the nuclear family which includes friends, neighbors, work associates, and significant helpers from churches, schools, social agencies, and institutions.

Related questions are: What influence does the source of help the family seeks have on the family? Is it appropriate? How important to the family are the "significant others"? How consistent is the pattern of managing in time of illness or crisis? Is this a source of strength in the present situation?

How individuals perceive the role of health professionals will influence the utilization and value they place upon the services of these persons. The past experiences the family has had with a community health nurse and the outcomes of its experiences will influence its expectations of her services. If, for example, its only experience was the help she rendered when a new baby arrived, or the weekly bath she gave to the grandmother, its knowledge of the scope of her services will be limited to these areas.

Why does the family think the community health nurse is visiting, and what does it think she can or will do? Community health nurses often fail to ask these kinds of questions and thus do not know how they are perceived by the family. In reality, however, these may be the most important questions the nurse can ask if she hopes to work with the family in developing a plan for nursing intervention. How do its expectations of the services it wants from the community health nurse coincide with the accepted functions? What is the difference between its perception of its nursing problems and the perceptions of the community health nurse?

The preceding discussion has dealt with the importance of systematic collection of a data-base about families in order for the community health nurse to define th health problems and identify the nursing needs. The kinds of information needed and the clues to be garnered from it have been pointed out. The analysis of this information for the identification of nursing needs is explored in the next chapter.

REFERENCES

1. See Appendix A of this text.
2. E. Duvall, *Family Development,* 3d ed. (Philadelphia: J. B. Lippincott Company, 1967), p. 8.
3. *Ibid., p.* 2.
4. R. V. Speck and C. L. Attneave, *Family Networks* (New York: Vintage Books, 1974), p. xxii.

BIBLIOGRAPHY

Ackerman, N. *The Psychodynamics of Family Life.* New York: Basic Books, 1958.

American Nurses' Association. *Standards of Community Health Nursing Practice.* Kansas City, Mo.: American Nurses' Association, 1973.

Anderson, E. M., Leonard, B. J., and Yates, J. A. "Epigenesis of the Nurse Practitioner Role." *Amer. J. Nurs.* 75 (October 1974):1812–16.

Becker, M. H., ed. *The Health Belief Model and Personal Health Behavior.* Health Education Monograph 2 (Winter 1974).

Becker, M. H., and Green, L. W. "A Family Approach to Compliance with Medical Treatment." *International J. Health Educ.* 18 (March 1975):173–82.

Black, Sr. K., "Teaching Family Process and Intervention." *Nursing Outlook* 18 (June 1970):54–58.

Bullough, B., and Bullough, V. L. "Poverty, Ethnic Identity, and Health Care." New York: Appleton-Century-Crofts, 1972.

Cowen, D. L., and Sharbaro, J. A. "Family-Centered Health Care—a Viable Reality?" *Medical Care* 10 (February 1972):164–72.

Duvall, E. *Family Development.* 4th ed. Philadelphia: Lippincott, 1972.

Hill, R. *Family Development in Three Generations.* Cambridge, Mass.: Schenkman Publishing Company, 1970.

Kaplan, B. H., and Cassel, J. C., eds. *Family and Health: An Epidemiological Approach.* Chapel Hill: Institute for Research in Social Science, University of North Carolina, 1975.

Kerr, L. "The Poverty of Affluence." *Amer. J. Public Health* 65 (January 1975):17–20.

Kirkpatric, C. *The Family as Process and Institution.* New York: Ronald Press, 1955.

LeMasters, E. E. *Parents in Modern America.* Homewood, Ill.: The Dorsey Press, 1974. Chap. 4.

Levine, M. "Adaptation and Assessment. A Rationale for Nursing Intervention." *Amer. J. Nurs.* 66 (November 1966):2450–53.

Mayer, M. A. "A Search for Assessment Criteria." *Nursing Outlook* 20 (May 1972):323–26.

McCain, F. "Nursing by Assessment, Not Intuition." *Amer. J. Nurs.* 65 (April 1965):82–83.

McCormack, G. M. "The Visiting Nurse Becomes a Nurse Practitioner." *Nursing Outlook* 22 (February 1974):119–23.

Milio, N. "A Framework for Prevention: Changing Health—Damaging to Health—Generating Life Patterns." *Amer. J. Public Health* 66 (May 1976):435–39.

Nye, I. F., and Berardo, F. M. *The Family: Its Structure and Interaction.* New York: The Macmillan Company, 1973.

Pollock, O. "A Family Diagnosis Model." *Social Service Rev.* 34 (March 1969):19–31.

Poston, R. "Comparative Community Organization." In Duhl, L., ed. *The Urban Condition.* New York: Simon and Schuster, 1969. Ch. 24, pp. 311–18.

Pratt, L. "Family Structure and Effective Health Behavior." In *The Energized Family.* Boston: Houghton Mifflin Company, 1976.

Presuvelou, C. "Nuclear Family Consumption: A Sociological Phenomenon." In Sussman, M. B., and Cogswell, B. E. *Cross-National Family Research.* Leiden, Netherlands: E. J. Brill, 1972.

Robertson, H. R. "Removing Barriers to Health Care." *Nursing Outlook* 17 (September 1969):43–46.

Speck, R. V., and Attneave, C. L. *Family Networks.* New York: Vintage Books, 1974.

Taylor, D. B., and Johnson, O. H. *Systematic Nursing Assessment. A Step Toward Automation.* Washington, D.C.: U.S. Government Printing Office, 1974.

Wilmer, D., and Walkley, R. "Effects of Housing on Health and Housing." In Duhl, L., ed. *The Urban Condition.* New York: Simon and Schuster, 1969. Ch. 16, pp. 215–28.

CHAPTER 7

ANALYSIS OF DATA AND IDENTIFICATION OF FAMILY NURSING NEEDS

Nursing has not as yet developed a specific conceptual framework that provides a theoretic base for the study of the health problems and nursing needs of families. Various concepts and theories from the behavioral, physical, and biologic sciences are being tested for their relevance to nursing. Some of the overall approaches used by other disciplines in studying families, which may have significance for nursing, have been summarized by Hill and Hansen[1] and elaborated further by Nye and Berardo.[2]

1. The *interaction approach* looks at the family in terms of the internal processes, such as role playing, status relations, communication problems, decision making, stress reactions, and socializing. Each person has a position in the family in which he perceives the norms or role expectations held by other individuals (or by the family as a whole) as the basis for his attitudes and behavior. In any situation the individual will define his role expectations primarily in light of their source and his own self-conception. Then he role-plays. The family is studied through analyzing the interactions of the role-playing members. The focus is on the internal structure of the family, with little effort made to view the overall institutional or cross-cultural relationships of family structure and function.

2. The *structure-function approach* views the family as a social system, and one of the many components of the complete social system—or society. Three major areas are emphasized: the relationships between the family and broader social institutions; the relationships between the

family and the subsystems; and the relationships between the family and the personality of the individual member. The family has functions to perform in society. It is composed of individuals who are significant for their functions in the maintenance of the family system, and ultimately the social system. Individuals contribute to the boundary maintenance of the system by acting in response to either the demands or constraints of the structure. The scope is broad and could include the interplay of the family and other systems in society, as well as the transactions between the family members. The emphasis, however, has been on the statics of structure with a concomitant neglect of change and dynamics.

3. The *situational approach* is based upon the assumption that all behavior is purposive in relation to the situation that triggered it. The individual reacts to the crisis or problem which the situation presents on the basis of how he perceives it and his previous experience in other situations. The situation itself, or the individual's behavior in the situation, is the focus for the study of families. By observing and analyzing this behavior in many situations, it is hoped by the students of this approach to eventually be able to understand human behavior and thus to predict it. The further development of this approach is not clear, as thus far the contributions have been negligible.

4. The *institutional approach* views the family as only one of the several institutions existing in society to satisfy personal and societal needs. Individual and cultural values are the main concern. The individual's values and learned needs are transmitted from one generation to the next within the individual family systems. These family systems and the cultural milieu in which the family exists make up the situation. Emphasis is on determining the impact of societal influence and other institutions on the family, with little or no recognition of the impact of the family on other societal institutions.

5. The *developmental approach* has as its focus the study of the developmental phases of the family from the wedding to old age, and finally the dissolution of the family through death. The changing developmental tasks and role expectations of parents and children, as they go through the family life cycle, as well as the developmental tasks of the family as a whole, are the basis for this approach. The successful development of the family depends upon how well each member meets his developmental tasks, and how clearly the family accomplishes its group tasks. This approach gives some idea of the family's vulnerability by its current developmental stage. It also allows generalizations to be made about the internal development of families, despite class, ethnic, religious, or other differences.

Kaplan and Cassel[3] have developed an epidemiologic approach to the study of the relationship between the processes of the structure and functioning of a family and its health status. The underlying theory is that susceptibility to a wide variety of disease and disorders is influenced by a combination of exposure to psychosocial stressful situations and the protection offered against these situations by adequate social supports. This approach seems to have relevance for health professionals in their work with families. However, further utilization of the method and refinement of the instruments are necessary before any generalizations can be made.

Recent findings in nursing research have uncovered some of the limitations in using conceptual frameworks from other disciplines in the development of nursing theory. There is a growing feeling among nursing researchers that nursing theory must come, at least in part, from the actual practice of nursing, and that it must be tested by actual nursing experience. Community health nurses, working with families in their own homes, have an unprecedented opportunity to be in the vanguard in identifying the processes involved in providing services to the family/group as a whole. In addition, they are in a strategic position to generate new concepts and/or theories about families, and also to add to the theories now in existence.

In this chapter each of the types of information collected about the family has been categorized according to whether it is most pertinent in:

1. defining the family health problems
2. developing the family nursing care plan
3. implementing the family nursing care plan.

This approach is not based on any one conceptual framework. It is, rather, a method of organizing the data in such a way that the relationship of the items to each other and to the family information can be clarified and better understood. The authors are aware of the pitfalls inherent in the analysis of the information in this way. However, we believe that by pinpointing the information most pertinent to the definition of health problems and nursing needs, to the development of the nursing care plan, and to the implementation of the plan, and by discussing this information in relation to each category, the usefulness and value of the data will be enhanced. The items under each category are shown in Table 3.

It has been mentioned previously that the steps in the nursing process are interdependent and that one or more steps may occur simultaneously. Similarly, the items and categories of the base-line information are not discrete entities in relation to the steps involved in the analysis of data. They are characterized by the interrelatedness of cause and effect,

TABLE 3. Family Information Most Relevant to Defining Health Problems and Developing and Implementing the Nursing Care Plan

DEFINING FAMILY HEALTH PROBLEMS	DEVELOPING FAMILY NURSING CARE PLAN	IMPLEMENTING FAMILY NURSING CARE PLAN
Accident hazards	Education	Availability and accessibility of health facilities
Current illnesses	Ethnic background and religious practices	Expectations of services of community health nurse
Demographic data	Health knowledge	Participation in community activities
Eating patterns	Health practices	Past experiences with health professionals
Food storage	Health problems as seen by family	Relationship of family to larger community
Living space	Health problems as seen by nurse	Role assignment
Medical history of each individual	Income and expenses	Role model of parents
Rodents and flies	Medical and dental care	Sources of help used by family
Sleeping arrangements	Pattern of decision making	Transportation facilities
Sleeping patterns	Relationships of members	Use of community agencies
Toilet facilities		Value system
to each other	Type of neighborhood	
Treatment and medicines	Use of leisure	
Water supply		

and cannot be looked at in isolation. At any one time the impact of an item or items may be greater in one aspect of the process than in another. The meaning of the interrelatedness of all the information in relation to the health of the total family and the resultant nursing needs is dependent upon the nursing skill, knowledge, and judgment of the community health nurse.

The items most directly related to developing the family nursing care plan are those listed in the second column of Table 3. bove.

The nursing care plan is the blueprint for nursing action in the family. It is based upon the nursing needs and contains the short- and long-range goals for the family that can be accomplished by nursing intervention.

The relationships of family members to each other, although they influence the definition of the health problem, have a greater impact on the kind of nursing care plan that is developed. For example, a family in which each member helps the others, and in which there is a feeling of family unity, requires a different kind of nursing care plan from a family in which these characteristics are not present.

How decisions are made in a family may be one of the key aspects of the nursing care plan. Too often, the decision-making apparatus of a family is bypassed in this step of the nursing process. The end result is that the health behavior necessary to meet the nursing goals is not sanctioned by the family and does not become operational, in spite of the efforts of the community health nurse.

The items relating to education, income, expenses, and the ethnic background and religious practices, while playing a role in determining health problems, exert a greater influence on the kind of nursing care plan which evolves. For example, the amount and kind of health teaching is determined by the educational level of the family; the ethnic background and religious practices also influence the kind and amount of health teaching that is necessary and acceptable to the family. The income and expenses influence all aspects and may be one of the more important determinants of the final plan and its implementation and outcomes.

The knowledge the family has about health, and the pattern of health practices are integral parts of the nursing plan. The core of the plan may be to correct some of the health misinformation and to change some of the health practices. The type of medical and dental care and the method of payment must not be ignored. The American people subscribe to the fact that good health care is a right of every individual, but the kind and amount of health care received often depends upon the economic status of the individual or family. What the family perceives as its health problems may not be what the nurse sees. These differences, if any, must be resolved as the plan is developed.

The type of neighborhood and its influence on the family also exert an influence on the successful development of the nursing action. The mores of the neighborhood, such as the upkeep of the dwellings, the way people view the police or other protective services, the waste disposal system, and the schools and churches, tend to force a general pattern of conformity on the families. The nursing care plan must be consistent with this pattern.

The items which are most directly related to implementing the family nursing care plan are those listed in the third column of Table 3.

Unless the nursing care plan can be implemented, the whole process up to this point becomes an intellectual exercise, or as some say, "an exercise in futility." The implementation of the plan is what the nursing process is all about—carrying out the nursing action based upon the identified nursing needs.

The items that take precedence in this step of the process are the ones relating to the resources the family uses in time of illness or crisis, its past experience with health professionals and community health nurses, and its expectations of services from the community health nurse. The information relating to these items gives many clues about the ability of the family to cope with its health problems and which situations will require outside assistance. The family's past experiences with health professionals and community health nurses color its expectations about the activities which can be carried out in its present situation.

The roles each member assumes and their appropriateness are important for implementing the nursing care plan. This is also true of the adult role models the parents present. It may be that the nursing action will require additional functions to be added to the current role assignments.

The value system of the family, a strong determinant of its behavior, exerts a strong influence on the implementation of the plan. This is also true of the items concerning the relationship of the family to the larger community, and its participation or nonparticipation in extrafamily institutions and organizations.

The availability of health and related facilities in the neighborhood, and the use and nonuse of these by the family, help in understanding this phase of the nursing process. The facilities may be utilized because of the prevailing mores of the neighborhood, but their accessibility is also an important factor. If people cannot reach the resources because transportation is inadequate, inconvenient, or nonexistent, the facilities will not be used irrespective of the quality of services offered.

IDENTIFYING FAMILY NURSING NEEDS

The steps in the nursing process are characterized by their interrelatedness, with no even flow from one step to another. The process is a developmental one, however, with each step dependent upon the other. The analysis of the data-base information to identify the family nursing needs is probably the most important step in the nursing process. The needs identified in the analysis form the basis for the ensuing nursing actions. Thus, if the needs are identified incorrectly, the remaining steps are meaningless, and the resultant nursing action may be ineffective or even detrimental to the family.

Throughout this book the authors have defined a nursing need as the contribution nursing can make to the solution of a health problem. In many sources today the terms "nursing diagnosis" and "nursing prognosis" are used quite frequently when nursing and the nursing process are being discussed. Although there is some beginning work being done on a diagnostic classification system[4] for nursing, there is not as yet any general agreement about the definition of these terms or of their meaning in relation to nursing. Each discussant uses them within his own frame of reference. Because of the confusion in the definition of terms, their connotation of disease conditions, and the lack of a nomenclature for nursing situations, writers have refrained from using them.

The data base about the family may be collected by the nurse or by any other member or members of the health team. The community health nurse, however, has the responsibility for determining what should be included in the data base; for analyzing the information to identify the health problems; and for determining the contribution of nursing to the solution, alleviation, and/or prevention of family health problems. Health encompasses the physical, social, and emotional well-being of a family and exerts a strong influence on its ability to carry out its functions.

The first consideration of the nurse is the analysis of the data to determine the family health problems. The nursing needs of the family are then identified from the health problems. A family or a community may have a health problem for which there are many nursing needs. On the other hand, there may be several health problems for which there are no nursing needs. The contribution of nursing to the solution of the health problem may take several different forms depending upon the needs of the family. For example, in some instances the nurse may help the family to cope more effectively with a present problem, while in another situation she may help to prevent a problem from occurring. The nursing will include such functions as anticipatory guidance, health teaching, health counseling, coordination, and referral, as well as direct nursing care. The nurse's primary focus is the prevention of disease and the promotion and maintenance of a high level of health for ultimate well-being.

The family information most pertinent to defining family health problems is shown in the first column of Table 1 above.

As discussed earlier, the data-base information about a family necessary to the community health nurse may be similar to that which is necessary for other professionals. However, the uniqueness of each profession lies in the kinds of questions each asks about similar data. In the following discussion the steps in the analysis of health-related data for the identification of family nursing needs are discussed, and some of the questions to be asked by the community health nurse are highlighted.

The steps in the analysis of the data directly related to health problems in the identification of nursing needs are to determine:

1. the relationship of the items to each other
2. the relationship of the items to the health of the individuals
3. the relationship of the individual's health problems to the family as a whole

4. the final determination of family health problems or potential problems
5. the contribution of nursing to the solution of the health problems
6. the statement of family nursing needs

1. *Relationship of the items to each other.* As has been pointed out, each item gives some clues about the possible presence of family health problems. However, it is only when the items are analyzed in relation to each other that the basis for a beginning understanding of health disequilibrium in the family becomes evident.

Clues about the presence of possible health problems can be garnered from these data. These clues also give leads to areas in which further investigation is necessary. For example, the demographic data, which includes information about the number of persons in the household, and their age, sex, and so forth, may indicate social or emotional problems related to overcrowding and lack of privacy. This item may also point out a problem of fertility or infertility in which family planning is a major need. Nutritional practices which contribute to health problems can be ascertained by the information about family eating patterns, and also the facilities it has available for the storage of food. The sleeping arrangements for the family and the sleeping patterns of each member are directly related to insufficient rest, and the resultant physical or emotional health problems.

The importance of the environment and its associated factors is taking on new significance today in relation to health and health problems. The home, although not an intact microcosm of society, nevertheless has many of the same environmental characteristics in relation to health. The amount of living space; the type of toilet facilities; the sources and amount of water available; and the presence of flies, rodents, and accident hazards are directly related to mental disorders, infectious diseases, food poisoning, rat bites, accidents, and lead poisoning.

The medical history of each family member and the current illnesses, including treatments and medications, are important items in the definition of health problems. The medical history not only points out past health problems but also indicates specific areas in which disease prevention and health promotion are necessary. The presence of acute or chronic illness in one family member is a key indicator of possible family health problems, as illness always has some effect on the equilibrium of the family and its ability to carry out its functions. Emotional, social, and physical health problems which follow a family pattern are also discernible from the health history.

Questions the community health nurse might ask to help clarify these relationships might be: What do the demographic data about age, sex and so forth have to do with the accident hazards? What is the relationship, if any, of the medical history to the sleeping arrangements or the living space? How do the facilities for the storage of food affect the eating patterns? Are the current treatments and medications consistent with the current illnesses?

2. *Relationship of the items to the health of the individuals.* After the effect of the individual items upon each other has been ascertained, then the data are analyzed to determine the impact of these relationships on the health of the individuals in the family. For example, what is the relationship of the current illness of any of the members to the medicines they are taking or the treatments they are receiving? The relationship between these two items may be triggering a health problem that has been overlooked. What is the impact of overcrowding and lack of privacy on the health of each of the members? It may be that no direct relationship can be found. On the other hand, it may be that some of the members are showing signs of stress, such as a change in sleeping patterns, that may be directly related to lack of an opportunity to have some private time or place of one's own. The lack of storage facilities for food may indicate that the food intake is inadequate to supply the necessary nutrients, particularly if someone is on a special diet for obesity or other condition. The impact of the environment and what it means to the health of the individuals should not be overlooked. There is much discussion today about the many factors in the environment which contribute to poor health, and of the necessity for identifying these factors in order to alleviate them or the stresses they generate. The health history and current illnesses of each member may indicate recurring themes which should be investigated further. If there is someone with a chronic illness in the household, he will inevitably have some effect on the family as a whole. The equilibrium of the family may be upset, which in turn will trigger a chain reaction of health problems.

Some of the questions the nurse might ask about these relationships are: What effect does the eating pattern have on the family member who has diabetes or is obese? What is the relationship of the sleeping patterns to the emotional development of the individual? What is the relationship of the pattern of family illness to the age and sex of the children? Answers to these and similar questions will help to clarify the health problems of the individual members.

3. *Relation of the individual's health problems to the family as a whole.* The health problems of each individual will have an impact on the family and may interfere with its ability to carry out its functions. For example, if a teen-age son or daughter has a drug problem, this will reverberate throughout the family. In addition, each family member will react in his or her own way, which in itself will be an added strain on the equilibrium of the family. The health problem of an aged parent will often be a

harbinger of a change in roles and relationships among family members. These changes may have implications for potential family health problems. Each family has its own inherent strengths and weaknesses, and each will react differently to the health problems of any of its members. Any change in one person will inevitably affect the group as a whole. This change can be the stimulus that causes the eruption of a latent health problem which might otherwise have remained dormant.

The analysis of these data will be clarified by such questions as: What family health problems are triggered because of the use of drugs by the teen-age son or daughter? Does the aged parent contribute to or impair the family equilibrium? What is the effect of the sleeping habits of the individual on the family sleeping arrangements and sleep patterns? It should be possible to state some tentative family health problems as a result of this analysis.

4. *Determination of family health problems or potential problems.* The tentative family health problems are further clarified, verified, or rejected, and new ones added by an analysis of their relationship with the other data-base information. As stated previously, all the information is characterized by its interrelatedness and cannot be looked at in isolation, although some may be more pertinent to one particular step in the nursing process than to another. Through the analysis with other information from the data base, the factors which contribute to the health problems will become evident, and other ones may come to light. For example, lack of money or health knowledge may be a contributing factor to the poor eating habits and resultant nutritional problems. Or the role assignments and relationships may be directly related to emotional family health problems not identified earlier. Questions pertaining to family health practices may help to clarify the source of a health problem, thus making it more amenable to solution. Through an analysis of the other aspects of the data base the identification of the tentative health problems will become more evident. This analysis may also bring other health problems to the fore which have been unrecognized. When the family health problems have been identified, they should be listed in order of priority. The increasing use of problem-oriented records by community health nurses provides a ready vehicle for the listing of family health problems. The problem list will also be adaptable as records become more and more automated.

5. *Contribution of nursing to the solution of family health problems.* As discussed earlier, a nursing need is the contribution nursing can make to the solution of a health problem. Therefore, family health problems, real or potential, are the framework within which family nursing needs are identified.

What is the contribution nursing can make to the solution of the family health problems? The community health nurse must examine this question very critically to determine the specific nursing contribution for each health problem. In the solution of some problems nursing can make a major contribution, while in the solution of others the possible contribution by nursing is negligible. For example, there is a fairly direct relationship between the alleviation of the health problems associated with the maternity cycle and the contribution of nursing in this area. On the other hand, the contribution of nursing to the health problems of dental care is less clear.

In this stage of the analysis, the proposed contribution of nursing should be listed opposite each of the health problems.

6. *Statement of family nursing needs.* The final step in the analysis is the determination of which of the family nursing needs the nurse should do something about. In this crucial step, she must look at the total data base for help in making judgments about the ability of the family to cope with its nursing needs. How the family has managed with past problems, the sources of help available to it, and the strength of the family as a group are some of the determinants which should be considered. The health behaviors of the family which need to be strengthened, those which need to be changed, and those which should be left alone are factors which must be considered in this stage of the analysis. A family member, a neighbor, or another health professional may be adequately meeting some of the nursing needs; thus, these needs should be left alone.

From this critical analysis will come the final statements of family nursing needs. From these statements, the nursing actions to meet the needs will be derived.

In this chapter, the data base about the family has been categorized according to the items directly related to defining the family health problems, to developing the family nursing plan, and to implementing it. Clues to be kept in mind in relation to each item were discussed briefly.

The steps in the analysis of the data to determine family nursing needs were outlined. A nursing need was defined as the contribution of nursing to the solution of a health problem. In the mid-seventies, a time of increasingly sophisticated technology, rapidly changing health delivery systems, expanding health teams, and strong societal forces, it is imperative that the community health nurse clearly understand her contribution to the health of families in order to make sound professional judgments about their nursing needs. The utilization of the nursing needs in the development of the family plan of care is explored in the next chapter.

REFERENCES

1. R. Hill and D. Hansen, "The Identification of Conceptual Frameworks Utilized in Family Study" *Marriage and Family Living* 22 (November 1960): 229–311.
2. F.I. Nye and F.M. Berardo, *Emerging Conceptual Frameworks in Family Analysis* (New York: The Macmillan Company, 1966).
3. B.H. Kaplan and J.C. Cassel (eds), *Family and Health: An Epidemiological Approach* (Chapel Hill: Institute for Research in Social Science, University of North Carolina, 1975).
4. Sr. Callista Roy, "A Diagnostic Classification System for Nursing," *Nursing Outlook* 23 (February): 90–94.

BIBLIOGRAPHY

Abruzzese, R. "The Nursing Process and the Problem-Oriented System." In National League for Nursing. *The Problem-Oriented System—A Multidisciplinary Approach.* New York: National League for Nursing, 1974.

American Nurses' Association. *Standards of Community Health Nursing Practice.* Kansas City, Mo.: American Nurses' Association, 1973.

Aradine, C. R., and Guthneck, M. "The Problem-Oriented Record in a Family Health Service. *Amer. J. Nurs.* 74 (June 1974):1108–12.

Bourgeois, M. J. "The Special Nurse Research Fellow: Characteristics and Recent Trends." *Nurs. Res.* 24 (June 1975):184–88.

DeYoung, C. "Nursing's Contribution in Family Crisis Treatment." *Nursing Outlook* 16 (February 1968):60–62.

Gebbie, D., and Levin, M. A. "Classifying Nursing Diagnoses." *Amer. J. Nurs.* 74 (February 1974):250–53.

Goode, W. "The Sociology of the Family—Horizons in Family Theory." In Merton, R., *et al., Sociology Today: Problems and Prospects.* New York: Harper & Row, 1965, Ch. 7, 178–96.

Helvie, C., Hill, A., and Bambino, C. "The Setting and Nursing Practice." Part II. *Nursing Outlook* 16 (September 1968):35–38.

Hill, R., and Hansen, D. "The Identification of Conceptual Frameworks Utilized in Family Study." *Marriage and Family Living* 22 (November 1960):299–311.

Kantor, D., and Lehr, W. *Inside the Family.* San Francisco: Jossey-Bass Publishers, 1975.

Kaplan, B. H., and Cassel, J. C., eds. *Family and Health: An Epidemiological Approach.* Chapel Hill: Institute for Research in Social Science, University of North Carolina, 1975.

Kluckholm, R. "Family Diagnosis." *Social Casework* 39 (February–March 1958): 63–72.

Matthis, E. "The Problem-Oriented System in Public Health Nursing." In National League for Nursing. *The Problem–Oriented System—A Multidisciplinary Approach*. New York: National League for Nursing, 1974.

Mundinger, M. O., and Jauron, G. D. "Developing a Nursing Diagnosis." *Nursing Outlook* 23 (February 1975):94–98.

National League for Nursing. *The Problem Oriented System in a Home Health Agency—A Training Manual*. New York: National League for Nursing, 1975.

Nye, F. I., and Berardo, F. M. *Emerging Conceptual Frameworks in Family Analysis*. New York: The Macmillan Company, 1966.

Roy, Sr. C. "A Diagnostic Classification System for Nursing." *Nursing Outlook* 23 (February 1975):90–94.

Schlotfeldt, R. "Research in Nursing and Research Training for Nurses: Retrospect and Prospect." *Nurs. Res.* 24 (May–June 1975):177–83.

Schwartz, D., Henley, B., and Leitz, L. *The Elderly Ambulatory Patient: Nursing and Psychosocial Needs*. New York: The Macmillan Company, 1964.

Thompson, S. P. "The Problem Oriented System in Home Health Agencies." In National League for Nursing. *The Problem Oriented System—A Multidisciplinary Approach*. New York: National League for Nursing, 1974, pp. 55–64.

Wald, R., and Leonard, R. "Towards Development of Nursing Practice Theory." *Nurs. Res.* 13 (Fall 1964):309–13.

CHAPTER 8

Developing the Family Nursing Care Plan

The nursing needs of families that have been identified by the community health nurse form the basis for the development of a nursing care plan. The nursing care plan is the blueprint which gives direction to the nursing intervention that ensues. It consists of the specific nursing goals for the family and the specific nursing action needed to reach the goals. The importance of the mutual dependence of the goals and the actions must not be underestimated. The clear statement of the goals for nursing intervention in the family makes purposive nursing activity possible. In other words, if the nursing goals are not clear, it really does not make much difference what activities the nurse performs because she does not know where she is going anyway. It is similar to a person who wants to go on a trip but does not know where he wants to go, so he takes the first means of transportation that is available. It will not make any difference what means of transportation he selects, as he does not know where he is going anyway. The nursing action to meet the goals also must be clearly stated; otherwise, the nursing activity may or may not be directed to the goals and becomes purposeless. There may be several nursing actions that can be taken, just as there may be many means of transportation for someone going on a trip, but the selection of activities must be clearly stated and be goal directed. The statements of nursing goals and of nursing action are dependent upon an accurate identification of nursing needs. If these are not identified accurately, the resultant nursing goals and actions will have limited results and could have an adverse effect on the family in its movement toward a high level of well-being. The community health nurse, because of her education and experience, must assume the responsibility and the concomitant accountability for identifying the nursing needs of families and for developing the nursing care plan based on those needs.

The nursing needs of the family as a whole are the central focus, although each family member has an effect on and is affected by the plan which evolves. Much of the nursing intervention may be directed at one individual, but the overall purpose is to improve the functioning of the family as a unit. Working with the individuals is one way this purpose can be achieved. The relationships of the individual to the total health of the family has some of the same elements that are found in the relationship of the family to the total health of the community. Just as the health of the family is reflected in the health of the community, the health of the individual is reflected in the health of the family.

In determining the nursing care plan some of the basic assumptions about the practice of community health nursing must be kept in mind. One of these is that the family has the right and responsibility to make its own decisions. Another is that the community health nurse works with the family in determining its health problems, in developing the plan of action, and in evaluating the outcomes. These assumptions make it clear that the active involvement of the family with the community health nurse, in mutually identifying its needs and planning the nursing action, is essential in community health nursing practice. People themselves are the ones who make their own problems and they also have the ability to solve them. To do this they must have correct and adequate information to make sound decisions. They also must be involved early in the decision-making process and in any plans which are developed. We all know of many laudable plans which have been developed but have died an early death because the people who were to be affected most by the plans were not consulted or involved as they were being developed. The early involvement of the family in the decision-making process is as applicable for the community health nurse as she works with her families as it is in all other endeavors in the life of the people. Unless the nurse really believes in the ability of people to solve their own problems, she will be ineffective in her nursing practice with families.

Community health nursing has a long history of working with families and with lay persons in developing nursing services. One of its basic assumptions is that people in the community are indispensable in all phases of the community health nursing program. The experiences and commitment of community health nurses to this assumption are particularly pertinent at the present time, with the demands by consumers of all kinds for control of the services they receive. These demands by the consumers are having a profound effect on professional workers in all areas. The education and experience of professional persons, for the most part, have not prepared them to participate with the consumers as colleagues in the decision-making process about the kind and quality of professional services to be rendered. As a result, no precedents have been established that can be used as guidelines, and there is much confusion by consumers and professionals alike about who has what responsibility and authority. Reaction on the part of the professional workers has been varied. Some have withdrawn completely and ignored the demands, an action which has tended to increase the tension from all sides. Others have abdicated their professional responsibility, with the consumer making all of the decisions, an action which also tended to increase the tension and conflict. Others, as in the long tradition of community health nursing of working with lay persons, are developing a partnership with consumer groups in which the knowledge of the professional and the needs of the consumer are shared, and mutually acceptable decisions are made about the kind and quality of services to be offered.

There is no doubt about the fact that a new era of consumer participation is in the offing which will markedly change the traditional patterns of providing services of all types to people. Out of this, either new and more relevant roles for the existing professions must emerge, or new professions will evolve to meet the demands.

Nursing practice, as was discussed in Chapter 5, has adhered closely to the medical model in which all information about the patient is directed to the physician, who in turn makes the decisions regarding the services that should be rendered. With this model the professional worker, especially the physician, has more information about the patient than the patient, who is to receive the services, has about himself. This model, which does not include involvement of people in making their own decisions, is no longer relevant for the individual, the family, or the community.

The family and its needs are the focus of a community health nurse. The family must make its own decisions about the nursing services that it needs, wants, and will use. However, it cannot make these decisions and understand the implications of alternate choices unless it has adequate and correct information. The family model, in which all the information about the family is directed to the family so that it may make sound decisions about the services it receives, is the operating model for the community health nurse. The family provides the nurse with information about the family situation, and the nurse provides the family with professional knowledge and information. Each in this sense is the expert in his respective role. This information is then pooled and mutual decisions are reached about services to be rendered. This kind of collaborative relationship strengthens the role of the community health nurse—rather than diminishing it, as some nurses fear—by forcing her to clearly identify the contribution nursing can make and interpreting this to the family. The contributions, or goals, of nursing differ from those of other disciplines, although they may have similar roles and functions. Herein lies the uniqueness of nursing!

As was discussed in the previous chapter, some of the data-base information needed about a family is more pertinent in developing the nursing plan of care and must be considered in this phase of the nursing process. These items are:

1. education
2. ethnic and religious practices
3. health knowledge
4. health practices
5. health problems as seen by family
6. health problems as seen by nurse
7. income and expenses
8. medical and dental care
9. method of payment for medical and dental care
10. patterns of decision making
11. relationship of members to each other
12. type of neighborhood
13. use of leisure

The knowledge, judgment, and sensitivity of the community health nurse is of paramount importance in the value and use of this information in the development of the nursing care plan.

The steps in the process of its development include:

1. determining the relationship of the nursing need to other needs in the family
2. establishing the priority of nursing need
3. establishing the nursing goals
4. determining the nursing action to meet the goals

Evaluation is inherent in each of these steps.

THE RELATIONSHIP OF NURSING NEEDS TO OTHER FAMILY NEEDS

Families, like communities, have multiple needs. These cover many areas and include social, religious, cultural, economic, recreation, health, employment, housing, education, and nursing needs, to name a few. These needs are constantly vying for attention, with both the internal and external forces operating in the family at any one time setting the stage for this drama.

The nursing needs must be looked at in relation to the other needs of the family. Nursing and health may be high on the priority list and occupy center stage, or it may be at the bottom of the list and not even be waiting in the wings. However, no one category of need has the same priority all the time; either because the need has been met for the time being or because other events have occurred, such as illness of the breadwinner, making a reshuffling of priorities necessary. In developing the nursing care plan the community health nurse has to keep these facts in mind, and determine the relationship of the nursing needs to the other needs in the family. It may be that the nursing needs cannot be met until a job is found for the husband, or that before anything can be done about improving the nutritional status of the family, marital problems have to be resolved. The value system of the family, which is a powerful determinant of its behavior, is a decisive factor to be considered in determining the hierarchy of needs and the relation of nursing to this hierarchy.

PRIORITY OF NURSING NEEDS

The nursing needs, in turn, have their own priority which must be established before the nursing action can be planned. Matching the nursing needs with the pertinent data-base information which was collected about the family, and with the available resources in the family and the community, will help determine the relative importance of each need and how best to meet it. Part of this process includes a determination of the strengths and weaknesses in a family. Families are generally much more aware of their weaknesses than of their strengths. Invariably, however, the strengths far outweigh the weaknesses, and it behooves the community health nurse to ascertain and exploit the strengths the family has. It also has some potential strengths which may have been lying dormant because there had been no opportunity available for their use. This knowledge, plus the data-base information collected relating to how the family has managed before in similar situations, or when faced with a stressful or crisis situation, will enable the community health nurse to make a judgment about the family's ability to cope with its health problems and nursing needs.

The relative importance of each nursing need and the plan to meet it also depend upon the relationship of the nursing needs to other pertinent information about the family. The educational level and the coping ability of the family will have a direct bearing on the amount of information to include in the nursing plan, and the method of teaching to be used. The relationships within the family not only help to clarify further the coping ability of the family, but also give some ideas about the kind of support and mutual help that is available.

One of the purposes of nursing intervention in the family is to increase its knowledge about health and to help change some of its health practices. The nursing needs are directly related to these areas, and the relationship between health knowledge and health practices must be ascertained. Correcting any misinformation or myths held by family regarding health may have to be the first step in nursing intervention before any other results can be obtained. Health practices, although not necessarily related to health knowledge, can be influenced by a greater awareness of current family health knowledge and provide an opportunity to explore alternative choices. Health knowledge and practices are also closely allied to the educational level of the family and how it gets information about health. The amount of information one obtains through reading tends to increase as one's educational level rises. Persons who utilize television and the radio as their main sources of information tend to be less well-informed than the "readers." The ethnic heritage and religious background of a family has a tremendous influence on its health practices. The kind of food, how it is cooked, and when it is eaten are related to the ethnic and cultural heritage as well as to religious beliefs and customs. Other practices, such as the role of women, decision making, discipline, and permissible social behavior are related to both the cultural and religious beliefs. These family practices have an effect on the overall health of the family and in turn influence the priority that will be given to the nursing needs. The most important nursing need may be given a low priority by the family because it is in direct conflict with cultural and religious practices.

There is no one pattern that determines what individuals or families perceive as their health problems and needs. Vickers[1] mentions that much depends upon the degree to which the individual seeks either to preserve an internal or external relation which he needs, or thinks he needs, or to escape a threat to a relation which will strain it beyond repair. The first he describes as goal-seeking—the successful completion of a goal in which the individual then decides whether the goal was worth seeking. The latter he defines as threat-avoiding—the successful avoidance of a threat so that the individual never has the opportunity of experiencing it and never knows if it was worth avoiding. These two approaches of goal-seeking or threat-avoiding are strong forces operating in a family when it attempts to determine its health problems. The health problems as seen by the family may be based on knowledge and sound logic, or they may be the result of long-standing practices and superstitions which have been passed down from generation to generation. The community health nurse must understand what the family believes its health problems to be and the basis for its belief. The priority of nursing needs will be directly affected by the intensity with which family problems are perceived.

The health problems as seen by the family may be different from those seen by the nurse. This is not unique to community health nursing, as there is always a gap between the knowledge and understandings professional workers have about health and those held by the consumers. However, in establishing the priority of nursing needs the community health nurse must recognize that this gap may exist and work with the family to resolve the differences. By keeping the family and its health problems the major reason for her services, the nurse narrows the gaps in perception and clarifies the priority of nursing needs. The improvement of the overall health status of the community is the ultimate aim of community health nursing, with the family as the vehicle through which this is accomplished. Therefore, the nursing services provided by the community health nurse are directly related to the health problems and priorities which have been established by the community. The priority of nursing needs in the family will not necessarily be the same as the priorities of the larger community. However, the nursing needs will be influenced by the priorities and by the accepted behaviors which are sanctioned by the community.

As can be seen by the foregoing discussion, the nursing needs of a family are only one small part of the whole constellation of family needs. In each family the priority of needs will depend upon many factors which influence the place of health in the hierarchy of needs. Similarly, the identified nursing needs will also have a priority of their own and will be based upon many of the same factors that determine the priority of other needs in the family.

ESTABLISHING NURSING GOALS

The development of the nursing care plan can begin to take shape after the priority of nursing needs has been established. This is a joint venture, with the nurse and the family working closely together in all phases. The choice of which individual or individuals in the family will participate is dependent upon the family decision-making pattern and how final decisions are made.

The plan, even though it is developed jointly with the nurse and the family, must be one that will be adhered to by the family. It may have been developed in a time of crisis, and when the crisis no longer seems imminent the plan may be abandoned. Or the plan may require too high a degree of commitment of the family over a long period of time, a commitment which it is not ready to accept and carry through. The acceptability of the plan in the neighborhood must also be taken into consideration. It must be congruent with the sanctions imposed by the neighborhood if it is to be adhered to. For example, if the plan involves a change in the sleeping patterns of the family that is in conflict with those of the neighborhood, the value of this change for the family should be weighed against the misunderstanding and disapproval of the neighborhood.

The effect of the plan on the family as a whole is another consideration. What changes in the assigned roles of each individual are necessary, and will this have a positive or negative influence? If, because of the illness of the mother, a 14-year-old daughter has to assume the homemaking responsibilities, what effect will this have on the daughter and on the family? On the other hand, one of the nursing goals may be to strengthen the family by more appropriate role assignments; thus, the role changes may be disruptive at first, but the long-range outcomes will contribute to the level of functioning of the family as a unit.

Are the necessary resources available in the neighborhood to carry out the plan, and what is the reaction of the people to their use? As was discussed previously, adequate facilities may be available in a community, but they may not be used because of misconceptions by the people about the services or because lack of transportation makes them inaccessible. If the resources are not available in the neighborhood, where can they be found? Is transportation available, and how can it be arranged? Long waiting lists for admission to hospitals and other health care facilities are not unusual today. How does this affect the nursing care plan? What are the alternatives to being at the bottom of a long waiting list?

The financial cost to the family, and what this means to the total budget, is a major consideration. The costs and charges of nursing visits from home health agencies, as with all other health services, are soaring. Even though the American people have agreed that health is the right of each individual citizen, and legislation has been passed to help to realize this ideal, the quality of health care received by individuals is still closely related to their ability to pay for it.

The source of medical care for the family will influence the development of the nursing care plan. The method of payment for medical care has some bearing on the source of care. If the local druggist is the source of much of the medical information, with the hospital emergency room as a last resort, how a plan which includes regular visits to a physician will be adhered to by the family must be considered.

One of the overall purposes of community health nursing is to help families help themselves. The movement of a family from dependency to independence is inherent in this purpose and should be reflected in the nursing care plan. In this movement, however, it should be kept in mind that contrary to popular thought, independence is not always a virtue and dependency is not always a vice. It may be as important to help a person to be dependent as to be independent. The autonomous nuclear family of today is much more dependent upon extrafamilial institutions and other resources than ever before. In order to fulfill its functions as a family it must know what facilities are available and how to use them. In this sense they may have to learn that some dependence is essential to optimal family functioning. By the same token, the highly independent individual who has had a myocardial infarction must learn to have a degree of dependence if he wishes to live out his normal lifespan.

The heart of the nursing care plan is transposing the nursing needs into realizable goals. This, as in all the other phases, is a joint venture which involves both the family and the nurse, with the family situation and its needs as the axis around which the nursing goals are defined. Family nursing goals give direction to the ensuing nursing actions and provide criteria for evaluating the outcomes. The goals are the road or path which the community health nurse travels in helping families solve their health problems to enable them to function at their highest possible level. The level of family functioning is one indicator of its health status.

The statement of nursing goals should indicate the health behaviors or observable facts in the family's ability to promote and maintain health and to prevent disease. The family and what it can do, rather than the nurse and what she does, is the main focus of the stated goals. For example, a goal which states, "To increase the family's understanding of budgeting," gives some idea about what the nurse will do, but does not indicate in any way what the family will be able to do. The same goal stated in behavioral terms might be "Husband and wife plan budget together," or "The budget is made out weekly," or "Each family member who contributes to the income participates in decisions about the budget." In these statements the emphasis is on the expected behavior from the family because of the nursing contribution. The outcomes can be evaluated through observation of changes in family behavior.

It is highly unlikely that the nursing needs of any family would ever result in only one nursing goal. Instead, they are more apt to fall into categories of goals. As the main focus of the community health nurse is on family health promotion, health maintenance, and disease prevention, the nursing goals can be categorized under these same headings. The completed statements will give a composite picture of the nursing goals for the family and will highlight the category in which there seems to be the greatest emphasis. Thus, it becomes possible to capture quickly the relation of one category to the other, to determine the short- and long-range goals, and to identify clearly the nursing action necessary to reach the goals. At the same time it provides the opportunity to pinpoint the highest priority of nursing goals and the timing of nursing action.

If the community health nurse is to categorize nursing goals under the headings of health promotion, health maintenance, and disease prevention, she must be clear about the nursing contribution in each of these categories. The nursing contribution can be defined as follows:

1. *Health promotion:* to increase the level of understanding and the expectations of health for the family. This may include changing or modifying health practices, increasing health knowledge, and developing understanding of normal growth and development.
2. *Health maintenance:* to maintain the family as a group in handling its health problems. This may include therapeutic nursing services, help in time of crisis, such as illness, birth, or hospitalization, and coordination of health and nursing services.
3. *Disease prevention:* to maintain and increase the level of immunization in the family to prevent the occurrence or recurrence of disease or illness. Level of immunization includes developing resistance to the social, emotional, and biologic forces which precipitate disease or illness. This encompasses such things as increasing knowledge about preventive measures in relation to specific diseases, such as special diets, breast self-examination, and vaccines; furthering understanding of the connection of the interpersonal relationships in the family with disease occurrence; and stimulating the family to participate in health screening and immunization programs.

With these definitions in mind the community health nurse can then translate the nursing needs into realizable nursing goals under one of these categories. Some statements of goals related to the expected family behavior under each of these headings might be:

Health Promotion

1. All family members have adequate sleeping arrangements.
2. The family eats at least one meal together each day.
3. Expectations of the children's behavior are appropriate to their age and sex.
4. Positive health knowledge is shared with friends and neighbors.

Health Maintenance

1. All family members participate in some way in caring for a sick member.
2. The family actively seeks help in time of crisis.
3. The family uses community health resources appropriately.
4. Each family member sees a physician for periodic checkups.

Disease Prevention

1. The diabetic diet is consistently carried out without disruption of family food patterns.
2. No family member is a scapegoat.
3. Each child has the necessary immunizations and boosters.

In determining which of the goals have the highest priority, the relationship of health promotion, health maintenance, and prevention of disease should be assessed very critically to determine the long-range impact on the family. For example, if most of the nursing goals are primarily in the area of therapeutic nursing services, what will happen to the family in the future if prevention and health promotion are neglected today? In determining the priority of nursing goals, the immediate and long-range outcomes for the family must not be forgotten. In some situations the long-range outcomes are more important and should have high priority, even if this should be more disruptive to the immediate situation. The knowledge, skill, and judgment of the community health nurse is of prime importance in this deliberation.

After the priority of nursing goals has been established, the next step in the process is to determine short-term goals which should be developed to facilitate movement toward the larger goals. The short-term goals give immediate direction for the nursing action and make it possible to have periodic evaluation of the nursing contribution. They also provide an opportunity to evaluate long-term goals and restate them if necessary. For example, one item under each of the categories will illustrate the selection of short-term goals.

One of the health promotion goals was, "The family eats at least one meal together each day." To achieve this may require changing completely the family eating patterns, changing the family's feelings about food, finding different ways of buying and cooking food, finding different food storage procedures, and changing the amount of money allocated for food. Each of these changes can be stated as expected family behaviors, and the outcomes can be observed and evaluated. For instance, let us assume that one of the stated short-term goals is, "The amount of money allotted for food is increased by 10 percent in two months." By the time this goal is accomplished and evaluated, it is found that one of the family members has a new job in which he works from 4:00 P.M. to 12:00 midnight for 5 days per week. Immediately it becomes obvious that the long-range goal of the family eating at least one meal together each day cannot be achieved. As a result it is evaluated and restated as, "The family eats at least one meal together on weekends," or "Family members whose working hours permit eat at least one meal together each day." Without the short-range goal with its built-in evaluation, the long-range goal might not have been changed.

One of the health maintenance goals stated, "All family members participate in some way in caring for the sick member." This may require teaching someone to give nursing care between the visits of the nurse, planning special foods, entertaining the sick member, relieving the caretaker so he or she may have recreation, changing the sleeping arrangements, keeping a supply of fresh linen on hand, and reallocating the budget items to meet extra expenses incurred by the sickness. In this situation a short-term goal may be, "The mother gives therapeutic nursing care between visits of the nurse." When this goal is reached, the evaluation indicates that the larger goal is still realistic and reachable, and progress toward reaching it is continued.

An example of a goal under Disease Prevention was stated as, "Each child has the necessary immunizations and boosters." Because of the family situation, it may be determined that this goal in itself is a short-range goal. The family already understands the value of immunizations, and it is only necessary to remind it of the time when they are due, to keep it informed of new developments, and at intervals to reinterpret their value.

As can be seen, there are many matters to consider in establishing the nursing goals. The key to making these goals meaningful is to state them in behavioral terms which can be evaluated. Three questions can be asked in evaluating the clarity of the statements of nursing goals. These are:

1. Are the goals acceptable to the family?
2. Is it clear where the family is going?
3. Can we tell when they get there?

If the answer is "yes" to all of these, then the nursing action to meet the goals can be determined.

DETERMINING NURSING ACTION

Once again it must be stressed that in actuality it is very difficult to separate nursing action from nursing goals, as they are often developed simultaneously. However, as has been mentioned many times. we believe that by breaking the various steps into small component parts the total nursing process becomes clearer and more easily understood.

The nursing actions necessary to carry out the nursing goals are easily discernible when the expected behaviors are clear. The category of the goal also helps to highlight the nursing action. The goals and nursing action to achieve them must be mutually agreed upon by the family and the nurse. The nurse has the responsibility of providing the family with sufficient and accurate information upon which it can base its decisions about what it wants to do and what it can do. The nurse must help the family to look at alternative choices and at their possible effects on the solution of the family health problem. The final decision about what nursing actions are acceptable rests with the family. As mentioned earlier, one of the basic assumptions of community health nursing practice is the right and responsibility of the family to make its own decisions. The importance of this assumption in this stage of the development of the nursing care plan cannot be emphasized enough. It is necessary that the nurse make sure that the family has all the available information and that it clearly understands the alternative choices. This is solely the responsibility of the nurse, but she must also support the family in whatever decisions it makes. For example, one of the nursing goals, with resultant nursing action, might be for the teen-age son with diabetes to give himself his own insulin, whereupon he refuses to accept this responsibility. The nurse should give him accurate and adequate information about the alternative choices to administering his own insulin, and their consequences to him in the future, as well as at the present time. The final choice rests with him. The community health nurse supports his decision and works with him in planning the nursing actions which are appropriate to the decision he has made.

The overall functions of the community health nurse in the family include direct nursing care, health teaching, referral, health counseling, anticipatory guidance, planning, collaboration, coordination, and health advocacy. Some of these are independent functions and some are dependent. The degree of independence and dependence is determined by each family situation. Bergman[2] has defined three levels of nursing activities by which she differentiates the independent and dependent functions of the community health nurse. They are:

1. *Assisting activities:* these facilitate the work initiated by another person who is responsible for the outcome. Examples are the nurse assisting a physician with a physical examination, or administering medications ordered by the physician.
2. *Complementing activities:* these are initiated by another person, but the nurse adds a specific nursing dimension for which she has responsibility. Examples are teaching a person with diabetes how to plan his diet which has been ordered by the physician, or planning and arranging for school health examinations.
3. *Initiating activities:* the need is recognized by the nurse who initiates action. Examples would be identifying nursing needs and planning the necessary nursing action to alleviate the need, i.e., helping the family cope with its health problems; or planning and conducting nutrition classes for obese teen-agers.

The nursing action to carry out the functions are many and varied. The same holds true in the choices of nursing action to meet the nursing goals of a family. Because of this, there are limitless opportunities for creative nursing actions which will enhance the family's ability to solve its own health problems. The nursing goals give direction to the type of nursing action, such as teaching, giving direct nursing care, anticipatory guidance, and so forth. However, the specific action and how it is carried out depends upon the creativity of the nurse as she works with the family in presenting alternative choices. To illustrate, one of the goals under health maintenance was, "The mother gives therapeutic nursing care between the visits of the nurse." The goal requires that the nursing action be geared toward teaching the mother to give the necessary care. However, how and what is taught will vary widely, depending upon the individual situation and what is acceptable to the mother and the family. This is where the creative potential of the nurse can come into full play.

The final consideration in planning the nursing actions is the estimated number of community health nurse contacts which will be necessary. How many home visits should be planned? Will attendance at group meetings, for example, parents' classes or the local Association for Retarded Children, alter the number of home visits? What kinds of information can be transmitted by telephone? How many contacts with other professional and nonprofessional workers on behalf of the family will be necessary? If it is impractical or impossible to provide the number of estimated contacts, what are the alternatives and what will be the effect on the solution of the family health problems? Are the estimated number and kind of visits consistent with the policies governing the community health nursing program, or should an exception be made for this family? Perhaps all the policies need to be reevaluated and changes made to meet the demands of consumers for more relevant services.

Evaluation of the nursing actions are continuous and ongoing. When changes occur in the family situation or in either the long- or short-range nursing goals, appropriate changes must be made in the nursing actions to coincide with the changed situations.

The component parts in the development of a nursing care plan have been discussed in this chapter. The identified nursing needs, which have been defined as the contribution nursing can make to the solution of a health problem, were the framework upon which the nursing goals and resultant nursing actions were built. Each step in the process of the development of the plan was discussed as it was affected by the family and as it affected the family. The steps were: determining the relationship of the nursing needs to other needs in the family; establishing priority of nursing needs; establishing the nursing goals; and determining the nursing action to meet the goals. The implementation and evaluation of the plan are the subjects of the next chapter.

REFERENCES

1. G. Vickers, "What Sets the Goals in Public Health?" *New Eng. J. Med.* 258 (March 1958): 589–96.
2. R.L. Bergman, "Public Health Nursing Functions: Assisting, Complementing, Initiating," *Nursing Outlook* 14 (July 1966): 42–43.

BIBLIOGRAPHY

American Nurses' Association. *Standards of Community Health Nursing Practice.* Kansas City, Mo.: American Nurses' Association, 1973.

Barnard, J. *Women, Wives, Mothers: Values and Options.* Chicago: Aldine Publishing Company, 1975.

Bell, R. "The Impact of Illness on Family Roles." In Folta, J. R., and Deck, E. S., eds. *A Sociological Framework for Patient Care.* New York: John Wiley & Sons, 1966.

Bergman, R. L. "Public Health Nursing Functions: Assisting, Complementing, Initiating. *Nursing Outlook* 14 (July 1966):42–44.

Braden, C. J., and Price, J. L. "Encouraging Client Self-Discovery." *Amer. J. Nurs.* 76(March 1976):444–446.

Buckles, J., Cashar, L., and Olson, L. "Learning Purposeful Nursing Intervention."*Amer. J. Nurs.* 68 (December 1968):2578–80.

Griffiths, E. I. "A Rational Approach to Patient Service Review." *Nursing Outlook* 17 (April 1969):49–51.

Harris, F. L. "Who Needs Written Care Plans Anyway?" *Amer. J. Nurs.* 70 (October 1970): 2136–38.

Helvie, C., Hill, A., and Bambino, C. "The Setting and Nursing Practice." Part II. *Nursing Outlook* 16 (September 1968):35–38.

Levine, M. E. "Adaptation and Assessment. A Rationale for Nursing Intervention." *Amer. J. Nurs.* 66 (November 1966):2450–53.

Mayers, M. G. *A Systematic Approach to the Nursing Care Plan.* New York: Appleton-Century-Crofts, 1972.

Mayers, M. G. "Home-Visit—Ritual or Therapy." *Nursing Outlook* 21 (May 1973): 328–31.

National Commission on Community Health Services. *Health Is a Community Affair.* Cambridge, Mass.: Harvard University Press, 1967.

Otto, H. A. "Developing Family Strengths and Potential." In Otto, H. A., and Mann, J. *Ways of Growth.* New York: Grossman Publishers, 1968. Ch. 9, pp. 77–85.

Palisin, H. E. "Nursing Care Plans are a Snare and a Delusion." *Amer. J. Nurs.* 71 (January 1971):63–66.

Pesznecker, B., and McNeil, J. "Relationship among Health Habits, Social Assets, Psychologic Well-Being, Life Change and Alterations in Health Status." *Nurs. Res.* 24 (November–December 1975):442–47.

Pratt, L. *Family Structure and Effective Health Behavior. The Energized Family.* Boston: Houghton Mifflin Company, 1976.

Sheridan, A., and Smith, R. "Family Student Contracts." *Nursing Outlook* 23 (February 1975):114–17.

Smith, D. M. "Writing Objectives as a Nursing Practice Skill." *Amer. J. Nurs.* 71 (February 1971):319–20.

Stewart, R., and Graham, J. "Evaluation Tools in Public Health Nursing." *Nursing Outlook* 16 (March 1968):50–51.

Tapia, J. A. "The Nursing Process in the Family." *Nursing Outlook* 20 (April 1972):267–70.

Vickers, G. "What Sets the Goals in Public Health?" *New Eng. J. Med.*, 258 (March 1958):589–96.

Webber, M. "The Prospects for Policies Planning." In Duhl, L. J., ed. *The Urban Condition.* New York: Simon and Schuster, 1969. Ch. 25, pp. 319–30.

CHAPTER 9

IMPLEMENTING AND EVALUATING THE FAMILY NURSING PLAN

None of the steps in the nursing process can be carried out as discrete, separate entities. At any one time there is much overlapping, with each step dependent upon and interchangeable with the other steps. This overlapping, dependency, and interchangeability is particularly evident in the planning and implementing phases, as implementation is inherent in developing any kind of plan. However, in order to understand more clearly the many facets involved in implementing the family nursing care plan, we have attempted to separate the two steps—but always lurking in the back of our minds are the pitfalls of this approach.

The nursing actions as discussed in chapter 8, which will help move the family toward reaching the nursing goals, have been identified mutually by the family and the community health nurse. The nurse has the responsibility for mobilizing all the available resources in implementing the actions. What parts of the plan must the nurse carry out herself, and what parts can be done by others? In answering this question she takes into consideration the roles and functions of other professional and nonprofessional workers, and their effect on the particular family and its health problems. The nursing goals for a family are different from the goals of other health professionals, but many of the functions of other workers are similar to those of nurses. In fact, the functions of all health workers have many similarities, with much overlapping and duplication. In addition, the roles and relationships of each health worker are very fluid and are constantly being revised. The degree of similarity in function and the fluidity of roles become strikingly evident when the family and its health problems are the focus of care. As a result, some of the nursing goals of families can be met by other professionals, such as physicians, social workers, or occupational therapists. Similarly, some of the goals of these workers can be met by the actions of the nurse. Families also provide a wide range of health care for their members. The actions of the family members are vitally important in the movement of the family toward a high level of well-being.

Increasingly, the multidiscipline health team providing comprehensive health services will become the pattern of health delivery for the majority of people. In these situations today, community health nurses are collaborating as full-fledged team members with other health professionals, and a peer-group colleagueship is developing. With the health problems of the patient and his family as the hub around which the team operates, the contribution of each team member is becoming more clearly defined for himself and for others. It is being cogently demonstrated that through this kind of approach new roles and functions emerge; at the same time the goals and contributions of each professional become more important and necessary.

Some of the data base collected about the family has more relevance to implementation of the nursing care plan than to other steps of the plan. As she implements the nursing care plan, the community health nurse should be constantly alert to how the following items relate to each other and to the total family situation:

1. availability and accessibility of health facilities
2. expectations of services of community health nurse
3. participation in community activities
4. past experience with health professionals
5. relationship of family to larger community
6. role assignment
7. role model of parents
8. sources of help used by family
9. transportation facilities
10. use of community agencies
11. value system

The community health nurse's responsibilities in implementing the nursing care plan include:

1. making decisions about carrying out the plan
2. providing nursing services
3. revising the nurse care plan
4. making referrals and collaborating with others in behalf of the family
5. coordinating the nursing and health services to the family
6. participating in continuing professional development

MAKING DECISIONS ABOUT CARRYING OUT THE PLAN

The resourcefulness and creativity of the community health nurse play an important part in how she uses the clues she garners from the available information as she moves into the decision-making phase of implementation. Data about the role model of the parents and the role assignments of family members help to determine what aspects of the plan can be carried out by the family itself, and the amount of support and continuous participation that can be expected.

The sources of help the family has used before should be examined, and their pertinence to the present situation ascertained. Perhaps the sources are still available and accessible to the family. At the same time there may be persons to whom the family members turn for guidance and whose opinions have a significant effect on the family. These persons, referred to as the *significant others,* are often overlooked by professional workers. As the nuclear family becomes more and more specialized, and as other family relatives become more dispersed, significant others, such as close friends, will play an ever-increasing role as sources of help and emotional support for families. Neighbors also have a bearing on how the plan may be implemented, although the role of neighbors, particularly in the impersonal environment of large urban areas, is changing as rapidly as every other facet of society. Speck[1] describes these significant others as part of the family network, and suggests that all these persons be included in any plan of care.

The values of the family and the emphasis it places on health also influence how the plan will be carried out. This is a particularly difficult area for the community health nurse, who often finds her values in direct conflict with the values of the family. The conflict may be centered around moral and religious beliefs, such as those concerning illegitimacy and abortion. Cultural differences, such as the use of practices that seem to contradict present-day scientific principles, often evoke conflict. Others, such as how the family spends its money, how it disciplines its children, and the cleanliness of the house, are less obvious value-conflict producers but can exert tremendous pressure when they are in opposition to strong beliefs held by the nurse. Working with families who have value systems different from her own does not mean that the nurse gives up her own beliefs and embraces those of the family. It does mean, however, that she recognizes the differences and guards against imposing her own values on families as she helps them to solve their own health problems within their own situation. This is consistent with one of the basic assumptions of community health nursing practice, that the family has the right and responsibility to make its own decisions.

As the family is the patient of the community health nurse, she must consider the effect that the presence of an ill member will have on the others in the family; and how the ill member affects the ability of the family to function as a group. In spite of some current thinking to the contrary, the family may not be the best setting for the ill member, and a more appropriate facility may have to be found. If he is to remain at home, the length of time the family can be expected to care for him and the kind of help it will need are factors to keep in mind.

The available health resources and facilities and how they can be mobilized will affect how the plan is implemented. On the one hand, there may be a dearth of facilities, and the nurse will have to determine how to get the necessary services. At the other extreme, there may be a plethora of facilities, and the nurse will be confronted with selecting the ones that will best meet the needs of the individual and the family.

Knowledge about the availability of transportation helps the community health nurse in making decisions about the most effective use of community resources. There is no one decision that applies to every family. In some situations it will be more beneficial to the family to have the health worker come into the home to provide the necessary services. At other times maximum benefits at lower cost will be achieved by transporting the individual to a community resource.

Who carries out what part of the plan will also depend upon the past experiences of the family with community health nurses and other health workers. Its past experiences will color the expectations of the amount and kind of nursing services it will expect and accept. This is also true of the services it will accept from other health workers. The consumer is becoming more and more involved in determining the kind of health care he wants and is demanding that the care he receives be rendered by qualified professionals. The lower-income segment of the population, in particular, is demanding that their neighborhood health centers be staffed by full-fledged practitioners. They are rejecting many of the services provided by less well-prepared personnel.

The relationship of the family to the larger community is also considered when deciding who can best carry out the nursing care plan. If the nursing actions are not consistent with current customs and values in the neighborhood, the family may lose face and become alienated from its neighbors. If the usual activities of the family do not include participation in social and health programs in the community, it will be more difficult for it to use the resources which are available.

PROVIDING NURSING SERVICES

The community health nurse weighs all the foregoing factors in making her judgments about who can best provide the nursing services needed by the family and how these services can be implemented.

In some instances it may be imperative for the nurse to provide the services herself, whereas in other situations she may supervise others who are providing it. An axiom for her to follow in making her determination is to ask, "What is the least preparation needed to carry out the nursing action?" She must keep in mind that manpower and talent are wasted if persons are providing services that can be done as well or better by persons with less preparation. Concomitantly she must be aware of the danger of assigning tasks that are beyond the training or competence of the person carrying them out.

If the functions require a high degree of skill or a special type of relationship, the community health nurse may provide all the services herself. She also may give the services herself in order to serve as a role model for others to emulate. In other cases, she may provide any of the services herself, in order to demonstrate or to teach someone else how to carry them out. In still other cases, she may elect not to provide any of the services herself, but will work with the other workers who are involved. In each instance, however, she retains responsibility for the quality of the nursing care the family receives. In asking herself what is the least preparation needed to carry out the nursing actions, she may judge from the data that the nursing needs of the family do not require the special skills of the community health nurse, but can best be met by a registered nurse. On the other hand, it may be that a licensed practical nurse has sufficient competence to carry out the specific nursing action. Or a home health aide, and in some instances a neighborhood aide, may have the requisite skills to meet the nursing needs of the family.

In making determinations about who can best carry out the nursing actions, the family members also play an important role. As mentioned previously, family members provide a great deal of health care and have a reservoir of untapped knowledge and skill in caring for each other which must be understood and utilized to the fullest.

The role of other professionals in carrying out the nursing care plan, which has been discussed previously, should also be exploited in behalf of the family. The community health nurse is responsible for the supervision of all persons providing nursing services to the family. The amount and kind of supervision will vary with each family and with the persons involved in the nursing actions. She serves as a consultant to other professional persons about the nursing needs of families and how they can be met. She also consults with other professionals when their specialized knowledge and skills are required for the family.

REVISING THE NURSING CARE PLAN

The community health nurse is constantly searching for new clues which will help her to have a better understanding of the family's health problems and nursing needs. In her search she may discover new relationships among family members, or new health problems unrecognized by the family. She also seeks clues from people outside the immediate family, such as other professional workers who know the family. In families where there are several other professional workers involved, she may initiate a case conference in which all the workers sit down together and share information in order to determine how best the total needs of the family can be met. Relatives can be a source for clues about the family and how they cope with health problems. How and why family members relate to each other and the role each assumes may be particularly puzzling to the nurse. As she observes and gathers clues from relatives about the life style and customs, the interaction pattern of the family members and how they relate to each other can be better understood. Neighbors and significant others are sources of further clues which help the nurse better to understand the family. How the health practices of the family relate to the mores of the neighborhood will increase her understanding about how best to meet the nursing needs of the family.

The family nursing care plan is designed to meet the nursing needs of the family and to help it move toward high-level well-being. The plan, to be effective, must be based upon information about the family. As new knowledge is obtained, the nursing care plan should be changed accordingly—in other words, the plan is a dynamic, vibrant tool that is responsive to new needs, rather than a static, self-contained instrument. Thus, the interchangeability and interdependence of the steps of the nursing process are demonstrated. Also, the necessity for constant ongoing evaluation of the nursing needs of the family, and of the nursing care plan and its implementation, becomes evident. The nursing care plan, and thus its implementation, will change as the family situation changes. Some of the changes, such as those that occur when a family member has an acute illness, will pinpoint the need for a change in the plan more dramatically than others, such as the garnering of further information about how the family members relate to each other. In both situations it is conceivable that the nursing goals and nursing action could change, as well as how and by whom the plan is being carried out. The judgments about the significance of the new information and its effect on the nursing goals of the family are a responsibility of the community health nurse.

To meet the changing needs of families today and in the future, it will be necessary to change some of the policies and practices that govern what kind of nursing services are delivered to families and how they are delivered. The working hours of agencies will have to be changed, new workers will have to be employed and trained, new relationships will have to be developed with other health workers, liaison relationships with other organized nursing services will be necessary, and coordination of community nursing services will be imperative.

MAKING REFERRALS AND COLLABORATING WITH OTHERS IN BEHALF OF THE FAMILY

In implementing the nursing care plan, the availability and accessibility of resources and facilities in the community must be kept in mind. The community health nurse has the responsibility to help the family benefit from the services of the available community resources and to interpret and clarify the type and kind of services that are available. Nursing does not have the competencies to meet all the needs of families and must be constantly alert to opportunities for referrals to other resources. Making referrals involves determining the extent to which nursing can alleviate the need in contrast to the possible contributions of other persons and resources. For example, a family member who has suffered a cerebral vascular accident may need to have rehabilitation services. The nurse may have to decide whether rehabilitative nursing services will meet his needs, whether a physical therapist is necessary, or whether he should be referred to a rehabilitation center. Her decisions will depend in part upon the community services that are available, but she must weigh all the alternatives as she implements the nursing care plan. If the patient receives only rehabilitative nursing care, will he be able to reach his full potential for rehabilitation? Rehabilitative nursing may help the patient resume the activities of daily living and permit him to stay at home, but is this the ultimate goal for the patient? If it is not, then the nurse will be doing a disservice to the patient and family by not referring him to a physical therapist or a rehabilitation center.

The amount and kind of nursing service that is needed must also be evaluated. For example, if rehabilitative nursing services can help the patient meet his full rehabilitation potential, how many visits are necessary, how often, and who can best provide them? If daily visits are required but only two visits per week can be made, what will be the final result? If the family and its needs are the focus for service, rather than the needs of the nurse or of the agency, these questions might be more amenable to a solution.

What happens to a family because of visits by a community health nurse? The nurses themselves can give examples of the value of nursing visits, but there has been no concerted, organized effort to document the value that has accrued to families because of the nursing input. At the present time there is much discussion but minimal action centered around the need for documented evidence of what happens to families as a result of service by a community health nurse. These discussions have accelerated as a result of some of the definitions of the levels of nursing care which have been developed by third-party payers. Many are geared primarily to the person with an acute illness and do not take into consideration the skilled nursing care needed for the surveillance and maintenance of the health status of individuals and families, or of the anticipatory guidance which is the armamentarium of the community health nurse. Unquestionably, many of the nursing needs of families visited by the community health nurse do not require skilled nursing care, and their requirements could be met with some kind of custodial nursing care. At the same time there are many families in the community who need skilled nursing care but are not receiving it. It is imperative for community health nursing to differentiate between the need for skilled and for custodial nursing care and to develop some immediate and long-range goals to meet these two kinds of nursing needs of people in the community. The plan must also include methods of reaching the persons who have nursing needs, but who are not receiving nursing service.

The entire nursing process, and particularly the implementation and evaluation steps, are positive action toward analyzing critically the contribution nursing can make to families and the outcomes of various nursing actions. The attitude of community health nurses has been that every family has some health need and undoubtedly could profit from nursing visits. This attitude, however, is no longer tenable in this era of dispersion of health manpower. Increasingly, community health nurses are going to be accountable for the value of their services and must bear full responsibility for demonstrating why their service to families is necessary.

COORDINATING THE NURSING AND HEALTH SERVICES TO THE FAMILY

The rapid rate at which new knowledge is emerging and the increasing development of technology are the major reasons for the need for specialists in all areas of endeavor today. Thus, we are seeing many persons who are highly skilled and knowledgeable in only one small area of a field, with little or no understanding of the field as a whole or of any of the other fields in which persons are involved. The health field, in which new specialists are appearing almost overnight, is a good example of this increasing specialization. Nursing, which has long been influenced by medicine, is also developing highly knowledgeable and skilled specialists. In addition to the increased specialization in the health field, each of the specialists has discovered the community and the family as his arena for practice. As a result, many specialists and specialized health services are available to the people. However, because of the uninhibited proliferation of personnel and services, there are many gaps, with few or no services available in some areas, and in others much overlapping, duplication, and wasted effort.

The community health nurse, with her education and professional commitment geared to the family as the patient, rather than to one age or disease category, can be called a "generalized specialist." She is in a key position to assume the role as primary care nurse to the family, to refer it to other specialists or specialized services as needed, and to coordinate all the health services for the benefit of the family as a whole. For example, when the needs of the family indicate that a specialist in psychiatric nursing or pediatric nursing is necessary for the alleviation of a specific problem, she refers the family member to the nursing specialist in that area. Or if the services of a social worker, nutritionist, physical therapist, and others are necessary, she refers the family member to these persons and resources. She then coordinates the services of the specialists and specialized services with all the other health services the family members are receiving as they relate to the total family situation.

In the early part of the century many nurses were employed by a variety of health organizations and provided a specialized service to people in their own homes. Thus, there were tuberculosis nurses, baby nurses, and communicable disease nurses, to name a few. Each had a special interest in one segment of the family and concentrated her efforts in that direction. Usually there was no communication between the nurses or coordination of the nursing services rendered, and the advice given to the family by one nurse often conflicted with that of another. By the twenties many of the public health nursing services to families were of this specialized nature. The effect on families of this kind of service proved to be chaotic, and it was imperative that changes be made. It was at this time that the idea of the family as a unit of service for public health nurses was conceived. As this concept developed, public health nursing services became increasingly generalized, with one nurse providing all the nursing services to the family. The specialized nurses in turn became consultants to the generalized nurse and helped her to utilize their specialized knowledge and skill as she worked with families.

Today we seem to be going through a phase similar to the early part of the century, with many nursing specialists providing services to families. Often these services are provided with little or no coordination with other services the family is receiving. In this context, for example, a mother who has had triplets—of whom one may be mentally retarded, one may have cystic fibrosis, and the third may be normal—could conceivably have three different nurses visiting her because of three different conditions. No studies have been reported about the effect of specialized, uncoordinated nursing services on families, but we all know of situations in which families have been disrupted and confused as a result. Other questions are being asked about what happens to a family when it must relate to many different professional workers.

The need for coordination of nursing services to families today is analogous to that of the early twenties. At that time, however, as the family became the unit of service for the public health nurse, it was possible to think of one public health nurse, with the help of specialized consultants, providing all the nursing services needed by a family. In today's society it is impossible for any individual to have all the knowledge and skill to meet the needs of families. Thus, community health nurses as well as other nursing specialists are being forced to define their particular area of competence. Nursing can no longer be "all things to all people." The focus must be on the health problems and nursing needs of the individual and the family and how these needs can best be met. The community health nurse, with her competence in the area of the family as a whole, must share meaningful information about the family with other disciplines and other nursing specialists; she must refer the families to whatever source can meet their needs; and she must coordinate her services with the other services the family is receiving.

PARTICIPATING IN CONTINUING PROFESSIONAL DEVELOPMENT

The community health nurse has responsibility for her own continuing professional development. In this era of rapid change in all areas of society, knowledge and skill can become obsolete in a very short time. DeCarlo[2] in discussing the effects of technology on our lives, has said that in a technologic society the emphasis is on knowledge, and that the future belongs to those who study for it and continue an attitude of lifelong learning. The necessity for keeping up with new knowledge and practices has been recognized by all health workers as well as by nursing. There is much discussion and some movement today toward requiring satisfactory participation in continuing education programs as a prerequisite for renewal of licensure for professional practice. Universities have established and expanded continuing education programs, professional organizations and other health institutions are intimately involved in continuing education for a wide variety of health workers, and full use is being made of technologic developments. Closed-circuit television, telephone conferences, films, videotapes, and programed instruction are utilized to provide educational opportunities for health workers to improve their professional practices and to keep abreast of new knowledge in their field.

In addition to pursuing continuing education programs, the community health nurse can keep abreast of new developments in nursing and in the community by such activities as membership in professional organizations, attendance at professional meetings, participation in institutes or workshops, reading of the professional literature, and involvement with other health professionals in case conferences, team meetings, and in-service programs.

Nothing can replace the knowledge and skill of the community health nurse in implementing the nursing care plan. How her responsibilities will be carried out and the emphasis given to each responsibility will depend primarily upon the needs of the family, the setting in which the nurse is employed, and the availability of other health team members. Irrespective of these considerations, the process will remain essentially the same.

EVALUATION OF THE NURSING CARE PLAN

Consumers of health care are demanding accountability with documented evidence that the health care professionals are rendering to them is producing the desired results. These pressures for constant evaluation are real and immediate for community health nursing, as well as for all other health workers. The competencies of each health worker are the hub from which his contribution radiates. Thus, the evaluation of the contributions each worker makes to solving the health problem of the individual, family/group, and/or community is one of the keys to the effective utilization of health manpower.

At present, evaluation of the quality of care consists of three approaches: (1) structure, (2) process, (3) outcomes. We shall give an overview of each of these approaches, followed by their application to the family as the patient of the community health nurse.

Evaluation of the structure includes such things as the setting in which the evaluation takes place. This is probably the type of evaluation with which those of us in community health nursing have had the most experience. It looks at areas such as the number of visits made per day, per month, or per year; the number of visits to a well-child conference, or to a tuberculosis or family planning clinic. If the number of visits increases over time, the increase is taken as an indication of the quality of care. This view is consistent with the American philosophy that "more is better." If, for example, an author publishes a large number of books, he or she is generally considered to be more successful than one who has a shorter publications list. Persons who earn high salaries tend to have higher prestige in society than those with a lower earning capacity. The more horse races a jockey wins, the higher his acclaim, and so forth. Also included under this structure are the number of nurses on the staff and their education. The more nurses who have additional education in community health nursing, the higher the quality of service—or so it is assumed. The organizational structure indicating how the service should be arranged and who is responsible to whom, also becomes important in this type of evaluation. During the fifties and early sixties, both public health and public nursing, in their preoccupation with how services should be organized and administered, were involved in this type of evaluation, although the structural approach was not used at that time. The kind and quality of supervision also comes under the rubric of evaluation of structure. Other time-honored phrases, such as "takes criticism well," "always neat and clean," "follows agency policies," "organizes work well," "writes records in the home," are all evaluations relating to structure. In the evaluation of structure, one has to make the assumption that these are the criteria which assure quality care.

Process evaluation can be classified as a means-oriented approach. It is concerned with the step-by-step procedures with which the practitioner carries out his/her responsibilities. The proponents of this approach to evaluation must assume that when the process is followed step by step, this in itself assures quality of care. However, we are familiar with the saying, "The operation was a success, but the patient died." This is a major pitfall of process evaluation in relation to quality of care.

Outcome evaluation is primarily concerned with what happens to the patient as a result of the services he received from the health provider. This approach can be classified as a goal-oriented approach. The emphasis is on the observable or measurable outcomes for the individual, family/group, and/or community. The adherents of outcome evaluation believe that it has value in identifying the contribution of each professional to the solution of health problems, and it pinpoints his accountability to the patient. One of the assumptions underlying outcome evaluation is that some elements of the structure and the process are related to the outcomes. However, the extent of these relationships is not entirely clear and needs further study. We have accepted outcome evaluation as the final step in the nursing process.

Each of the steps of the nursing process has provided opportunity for built-in evaluation by the collection of a data base, by the determining of the health problems from these data, by the identification of the nursing needs from the health problems, by the statement of short- and long-range goals in behavioral terms, and by the built-in evaluative mechanism in the implementation of the plan. The important factor in the evaluation, however, is in the statement of the short- and long-range goals. They must be stated in relation to what the family can do because of the intervention by the nurse—in other words, in behavioral terms. The family and its health problems become the focal point in this situation, rather than the nurse and what she does or does not do. Unquestionably, changes in the health behavior of families are greatly influenced by the imagination, skill, judgment, and knowledge of the nurse. But our main concern is the benefits that accrue to the patient and can be observed or measured. Utilizing the short- and long-range behavioral goals for evaluation makes it possible to systematically document areas in which nursing makes a difference in the solution of a health problem, and areas where it does not make any difference. Other benefits from this endeavor will be the identification of problem areas for further research, and the formulation of researchable questions.

If the goals were reached, we must ask additional questions. The first is, "Would the goals have been met without nursing intervention?" This is a vital question and gets at the heart of the cause and effect of nursing intervention. Throughout this book a nursing need has been defined as the contribution nursing can make to the solution of a health problem. This presupposes that in the early steps of the nursing process, family health problems and nursing needs were identified correctly. If, however, the final evaluation indicates that the health problems would have been resolved without nursing intervention, it raises some questions about the accuracy of the identified nursing needs. If it can be documented that the same nursing goals in other families under different situations have been met consistently without nursing intervention, appropriate changes should be made in community health nursing practices.

Another question for which answers must be sought is, "Were the outcomes which accrued from reaching the goals worth the effort, time, and money?" Would a little more or a little less effort or emphasis have made any difference? For example, one of the nursing goals in a family with a mentally retarded child may have been for the child to learn how to feed and dress himself. The nursing action included bi-weekly visits by the nurse. The evaluation could reveal that if daily visits had been made for the first 2 or 3 weeks, the outcomes could have accrued sooner, and at the same time the ability of the family to cope with the problem and to seek help when needed would have been strengthened. As a result, only minimal follow-up visits by the nurse would have been necessary. A critical evaluation of the amount of nursing service expended in relation to the value of the outcomes will provide some needed guidelines for setting priorities for nursing service.

In reaching the goals, were there any unanticipated outcomes, either positive or negative? It is inevitable that nursing actions in a family will lead to some unanticipated changes in family behaviors. An example of a positive effect is the following: A nursing goal is stated for an obese teen-age daugher to lose 15 to 20 pounds in 6 months. The daugher reaches the goal, and at the same time the diet and eating patterns of the total family improve. An example of an unexpected negative effect could occur from a goal which was geared to keeping an ill member at home. Because of the need of the ill member for a great deal of attention, the needs of the other members are neglected. As a result, signs of family disequilibrium appear, such as truancy from school and increased absence from the home. Evaluation of why these side effects occur will make the role of the nurse as an initiator of behavioral change more clearly understood.

If the nursing goals are not reached, the reasons must be ascertained. The reality of the goals for the family should be carefully considered. It may be that the ability of the family to solve its own problems was overestimated and that too much was expected from it at this particular time. As a result the nursing actions were inappropriate and tended to raise the anxiety level of the family. On the other hand, the goals may have been realistic but something happened along the way which changed the family's commitment to them. The clues indicating the changes in commitment were not evident or were not recognized.

The actions of the community health nurse provide the key to whether the nursing goals are met and give evidence of the contribution of nursing to the solution of family health problems. The value of the nursing care plan rests solely upon the resourcefulness and creativity of the nurse as she implements it. What about the nursing actions—were they relevant to the goals and appropriate for the family? The community health nurse must make these distinctions in each family situation. What effect did the timing of the nursing actions have on the attainment of the goals? Oftentimes the idea and the substance of an action is sound, but its effectiveness depends upon the timing, or how and when it was introduced and carried out. Did the nurse have the education and experience to provide the necessary nursing services, to make full utilization of community resources, and to understand the present and future implications of her actions on the family? It may be necessary to increase her competency in work with the family as patient through providing inservice education programs, opportunities to attend workshops and institutes, and by instituting changes in supervisory practices. How did the family feel about the nurse, and how did the members relate to her? The importance of the relationship the community health nurse establishes with the family cannot be underestimated. It is impossible for any one person to relate equally well with everyone. The community health nurse is no exception; she must be aware of this and of her effect as a person on the family.

Community health nursing has recognized the necessity for developing critieria to evaluate the quality of nursing services. Nursing administrators are experimenting in various ways with utilization reviews of patient records and with nursing audits. Accreditation of community health nursing programs is another aspect of evaluation. In addition to these administrative endeavors, evaluation must be included as a step in the nursing process and must become an inherent and viable tool for each community health nurse. Only in this way will there be documented evidence of the effectiveness of the contribution of nursing to the solution of family and community health problems.

REFERENCES

1. R.V. Speck and C.L. Atteneave, *Family Networks* (New York: Vintage Books, 1974), p. 6.
2. C.R. DeCarlo, "Perspectives on Technology", In F. Ginsberg, ed. *Technology and Social Change.* (New York: Columbia University Press, 1961). Ch. 1, p. 29.

BIBLIOGRAPHY

American Nurses' Association. *Standards of Community Health Nursing Practice.* Kansas City, Mo.: American Nurses' Association, 1973.

American Public Health Association. "Glossary of Evaluative Terms in Public Health." *Amer. J. Public Health* 60(August 1970):1546–52.

Becker, M.H. *The Health Belief Model and Personal Health Behavior.* Health Education Monograph. 2 (Winter 1974).

Block, D. "Evaluation of Nursing Care in Terms of Process and Outcomes." *Nurs. Res.* 24(July–August 1975):256–63.

Doster, D. D. "Utilization of Available 'Nurse Power' in Public Health." *Amer. J. Public Health* 60(January 1970):25–37.

George, M., Ide, K., and Vamberg, C. "The Comprehensive Health Team: A Conceptual Model." *J. Nurs. Admin.* 1(March–April 1971):9–13.

Gilson, B., *et al.* "The Sickness Impact Profile: Development of an Outcome Measure of Health Care." *Amer. J. Public Health* 65(December 1975):1304–14.

Hegyvary, S., and Deiter, R. K. "Monitoring Nursing Care Quality". *Amer. J. Public Health* 65(March 1975):284–90.

Hilger, E. E. "Developing Nursing Outcome Criteria." In *Nursing Clinics of North America.* Philadelphia: W. B. Saunders Company, 1974, pp. 323–30.

Jones, M. C. "An Analysis of a Family Folder." *Nursing Outlook* 16(December 1968):48–51.

Krumme, U. "The Case for Criterion-Referenced Measurement. *Nursing Outlook* 23(December 1975):764–70.

Lindeman, C. A. "Measuring Quality of Nursing Care." Part 1. *J. Nurs. Admin.* 6(June 1976):7–9.

National Commission on Community Health Services. *Health Is a Community Affair.* Cambridge, Mass.: Harvard University Press, 1967.

National League for Nursing. *Quality Assurance–A Joint Venture.* New York: National League for Nursing, 1975.

Phaneuf, M. C. "Nursing Audit for Evaluation of Patient Care." *Nursing Outlook* 14(June 1966):51–54.

Roberts, D., and Hudson, H. *How to Study Patient Progress.* Public Health Service Publication No. 1169. Washington, D.C.: Government Printing Office, 1964.

Ruano, B. J. "This I Believe . . . about Nurses Innovating Change." *Nursing Outlook* 19(June 1971):416–18.

Schwartz, D. R. "Toward More Precise Evaluation of Patient's Needs." *Nursing Outlook* 13(May 1965):42–44.

Speck, R. V., and Attneave, C. L. *Family Networks.* New York: Vintage Books, 1974.

Spradley, L. "We Care Enough to Come to You." *Nursing Outlook* 22(May 1974):168–81.

Stewart, R., and Graham, J. "Evaluation Tools in Public Health Nursing." *Nursing Outlook* 16(March 1968):50–51.

Walton, M. H. "Quality Assurance in Health Care." In *Quality Assurance Models for Nursing Education.* New York: National League for Nursing, 1976. pp. 27–32.

Wandelt, M., and Aget, J. *Quality Patient Care Scale.* New York. Appleton-Century-Crofts, 1974.

Wandelt, M., and Stewart, D. *Slater Nursing Competencies Scale.* New York: Appleton-Century-Crofts, 1972.

Watson, A., and Mayers, M. "Evaluating the Quality of Patient Care through Retrospective Chart Review." *J. Nurs. Admin.* 6(March–April 1976):17–21.

CHAPTER 10
THE COMMUNITY AS THE PATIENT

Community health nursing has a dual responsibility: caring for the family and, likewise, the community. Chapters 5 through 9 were concerned with the concept of the family as the patient. The focus now shifts to the other equally important patient of the community health nurse—the community.

Public health nursing early recognized the need to work with others in the community and with the community itself for disease prevention and health promotion. In the 1920s public health nursing was the standard-bearer for the improvement and expansion of health services to people. This same broad approach to community health is equally valid today; the situation, however, has changed. The concept of the community as the most fruitful arena for improving the health of the people, held for many years primarily by the public health team (nurse, physician, and sanitarian), has now been embraced by an ever-increasing array of health and health-related workers. The community has been given highest priority, and all eyes seem to be turned in its direction. It has become the focal point of interaction for the growing army of concerned and involved health workers and for the myriad new and expanding health programs. Community health nursing is a charter member of this growing group.

The goals of public health have changed and broadened over the years in relation to developments in medical science and technology, the social and political progress of the country, and the rising aspirations of the people. Early definitions of public health were concerned primarily with sanitary controls for the protection of the individual against health hazards with which he was unable to cope—such as unsafe food and water, and communicable disease. Winslow's definition of public health, written many years ago, is stated in such broad and flexible terms that it is still useful for today and the future:

> Public Health is the Science and Art of (1) preventing disease, (2) prolonging life, and (3) promoting health and efficiency through organized community effort for
>
> a. the sanitation of the environment,
> b. the control of communicable infections,
> c. the education of the individual in personal hygiene,
> d. the organization of medical and nursing services for the early diagnosis of preventive treatment of disease, and
> e. the development of the social machinery to insure everyone a standard of living adequate for the maintenance of health, so organizing these benefits as to enable every citizen to realize his birthright of health and longevity.[1]

A key phrase in this definition is "through organized community effort." If Winslow, often referred to as the father of public health, were writing this definition today, he would undoubtedly include the concept of comprehensive community health planning, since the age of comprehensive health planning is here and those who are concerned with health must accept it.

The need for programs for the protection of the people against the innumerable physical, emotional, social, and environmental health hazards is just as important today as it ever was. The need for comprehensive health programs for the diagnosis, treatment, rehabilitation, disease prevention, and education of the public for health also remains of vital importance. The health programs as a priority, however, have changed in relation to other problems. Poverty, partly the result of urbanization and industrialization, is one of the greatest contemporary problems and can no longer be tolerated in an affluent society. Changes in demography and life expectancy, and advances in medical science are just a few of the factors which have resulted in the high priority given to chronic disease programs and research. Environmental and drug problems are of vital concern. Health, however, is only one aspect of life. It affects and is affected by many other factors. Health needs emerge and change as society changes. They must be identified and accorded appropriate priority within the framework of the total community.

The most stable characteristic of the present health care system is change, characterized by expansion, experimentation, and confusion. Traditional patterns for the delivery of health care are no longer adequate for the twentieth and twenty-first centuries, although many health professionals have been slow either to realize or to admit this fact. We are in the midst of a health care revolution which has come about as the result of far-reaching and rapid societal changes and developments. To name a few: America as an affluent society can afford high-quality health care, and this is the right of all citizens, no longer just a privilege; a socially conscious people has declared war on poverty; increasing urbanization has resulted in an urgent demand for new patterns of health service; rapid technologic and scientific developments and new knowledge have made possible and urgent better methods of treatment and patterns of care; a better-educated and informed public knows what kind of care is possible and demands this care; more people are participating in decision making and asserting the what, where, how, and who regarding community health services; the lines between specialization and generalization are more sharply drawn, while those between care and cure are becoming blurred; and the federal government, increasingly sensitive to the social welfare needs of the country, has responded directly to the urgent demands of the people for better health care.

It is probably safe to say that never before in the history of our country have so many people been concerned about and involved in the community and its problems, including its health problems. No health worker today needs to be reminded of the proliferation of new, different, comprehensive, specialized, reorganized, or combined health programs. He is probably deeply involved in developing one himself. Comprehensive health centers, community mental health centers, storefront clinics, prepaid insurance group practice plans, outreach programs, to name only a few, are multiplying. Many of these new programs are creative and innovative and have resulted in broader and improved care. They have, however, also resulted in disruptions as well as gaps, overlaps, and duplication of previously existing services—and considerable confusion about who does what. At this point in time no one is quite sure just who is responsible for what. This uncertainty creates both excitement and frustration. There are no ground rules. There are, however, fewer people watching from the sidelines and more in the arena—the community.

Changes within the health system itself, always occurring, are accelerating with the emergence of new health problems, new knowledge, and an expanding health team. A major factor is the changing role of the government in financing and influencing both health planning and future directions of health care. The relationship between the health system and other community systems is constantly shifting, as national priorities of war, peace, economics, law, order, education, and health shift and change. The whole concept of national health has changed and broadened with positive health a goal; and a national health plan, still on the horizon, is nearer to becoming a reality. Not the least important is the change which has occurred in the consumer of health care. His aspirations for health are high. His knowledge is greater than ever before. He is tired of poor and expensive care, and fragmented services. He is demanding change, and will have it.

John Gardner, in discussing the Great Society, reminded us that, "Every great creative performance since the initial one has been in some measure a bringing of order out of chaos."[2] To bring order out of chaos is a major task of all who are concerned with health. Americans have the knowledge and the resources but have not been able or willing to implement a flexible, economically feasible plan of health organization through which quality service can be made available to all who need it. Our heritage of democracy and individualism, coupled with the complexity of an urban society, makes the task of planning quality care a herculean one. Whether this can be done depends more on our wisdom and intelligence than on money or words.

The word *community* is so frequently used today, in such a variety of contexts, and by people with such different frames of reference, that its meaning has become blurred and nebulous. According to Sanders[3] the community may be viewed in three ways—as a place, as a social system, and as a collection of people. Each has relevance to health.

The view of the community as a place is important for community health workers. Environment, housing, and transportation are all related to geographic location, as are population composition and distribution, health services, resources, and facilities. Statistical and epidemiologic studies are frequently based on data from specific localities or circumscribed communities. Of increasing importance to all health workers is knowledge of political and legislative jurisdiction, including census tracts and regions—all area-based.

A community can also be viewed as a social system, with its own pattern of interaction which has resulted from the interrelationship of many systems within the community. The community is actually a combination of all the social units and systems which have been developed to carry out its major functions. Sanders, in describing health as one of the major community systems, states:

> A major community system, whether it be education or the economy, has identifiable characteristics, such as (1) a structure, or a related series of agencies, organizations, or establishments; (2) a set of functions, both manifest and latent; (3) functionaries, or persons charged with the responsibility of promoting the interest of the system or major segments of it; (4) ideology or rationale, which provides the justification for the continuation of the system; (5) paraphernalia, or the necessary equipment and material resources for carrying out the expected activities; and (6) linkages with other systems within and without the community.[4]

Finally, the concept of the community as a collection of people is an extremely important one for health workers.

> The difference between the treatment of disease in an ill individual and planning for improved health for groups of people has been summed up clearly by Carl Taylor. Since the "patient" is a group, pulse and temperature readings are a series of statistical measurements: birth rates, death rates, incidence of particular diseases. Says Dr. Taylor, "Such indices require a basic readjustment in thinking. A woman is either pregnant or not pregnant; a community is about 3 per cent pregnant. A patient has or does not have heart disease; the community always has heart disease, though the rate may go up or down."[5]

A form of community exists wherever a group of people band together for their mutual protection and common good, or to buy and sell their services. The community, therefore, is in reality not buildings, organizations, or a geographic area. It is people—people who are transmitters of value systems and culture, of attitudes toward health and illness, and who vary in myriad ways as to ethnicity, social class, education, religion, and health. Klein defines community as

> patterned interaction within a domain of individuals seeking to achieve security and physical safety, to derive support at times of stress, and to gain selfhood and significance throughout the life cycle. . . . The definition rests on interactions of individuals rather than on social organizations whose nature and functions are a manifestation of those interactions. The term "domain" is used to refer both to a physical place that can be geographically located and to a social-psychological place (such as a community of interest) that is "phenomenologically real" to those who inhabit it. Community as viewed here, is not man's habitat; rather, it is man-in-habitat, for a habitat is not meaningful without inhabitants.[6]

This fact was graphically illustrated in a recent radio announcement to the effect that it is now possible to purchase, at a relatively low cost, an entire deserted town in a midwestern state—a town complete with houses and schools, streets and transportation, and other community resources. The forces of urbanization were too strong for this town. This is not a community. There are no people. Conversely, strip the inhabitants of a community of all the goods and services available and necessary to them, and they will not survive for very long. John Alexander provides another illustration in his description of Oshkosh, Wisconsin:

> A city is like a living organism. It has a shape and a form—a skeleton, so to speak, of streets, city limits, blocks and buildings. But a city is more than that. A city has life. It has people circulating, in,

> through, and around those features which constitute its skeleton. Without its people Oshkosh would be dead. To be sure, the streets would still be there; the factories, the stores, the schools, the parks would all be in their same location. Perhaps from the air it would still look like Oshkosh, but it would not be Oshkosh. It is the people who make a city. They constitute the life that ebbs and flows through the inanimate framework.[7]

Klein further emphasizes the importance of community as follows:

> This community, even in today's world of rapid mobility and urban sprawl, is a highly important habitat of man. For it is through community that man is fed and housed, seeks work, educates his children, and in a variety of ways maintains his safety and security. It is also through the community that man discovers problems and their solutions, finds spiritual sustenance, exercises his desire for significant participation in life, and occasionally achieves the highest levels of self-actualization and fulfillment.[8]

There are a variety of approaches which may be used to gather information about a community and contribute to an understanding of its dynamics. Communities, like families, have their own patterned interaction between individuals, families, groups, and organizations, which varies from community to community depending upon the characteristics, needs, and value systems of the population. It is not easy to capture this sense of interaction within a specific community. Communities have many similarities. All have people, all have physical facilities, and all have an ongoing government, business, and social life. But there are differences as well, among them, relative to size, physical facilities, and composition of the population.

For the purpose of this book, we have adopted Warren's definition of a community,[9] which states: "A community is that combination of social units and systems which performs the major social functions having locality relevance." In other words, this means that a community organizes the activities of society in order for people to have daily access to those broad areas of functioning which are necessary in day-to-day living.

The functions of a community, as defined by Warren, are:

1. *Production-distribution-consumption.* It includes the service activities of industry, business, the professions, religion, education, government, and so forth.
2. *Socialization.* It is a process for the transmission of the prevailing knowledge, social values, and behavior patterns to individual members. Schools are one good example.
3. *Social control.* It includes the group influence on behavior by demanding conformity to norms. Norms vary from community to

community. Government is particularly involved in this area, with courts, police, and so forth.

4. *Social participation.* It is accomplished through participation in religious and voluntary organizations within the community.
5. *Mutual support.* This function is carried out through social agencies, hospitals, health departments, and so forth.[10]

Earlier, we indicated that the community health nurse is a "specialized generalist." This is probably one of her greatest assets at the present time. Chang[11] suggests that because of this approach the community health nurse is able to work in a health team, to teach and encourage other workers, to communicate with and motivate population groups, and to interrelate community health nursing with other systems in the community, such as the educational, social, and cultural.

The community health nurse is the only professional health worker who has theory and practice in community health and community health nursing as part of her generic education. Thus, as a profession, nursing is better prepared than any other group to take leadership in the identification of health problems in a community and in mobilizing the people to participate in solving their own health problems. The sphere of action for community health nursing is and must be the broader community, rather than the program of any one specific agency. To participate as a full partner and to assume the leadership for which it is prepared, community health nursing must become more knowledgeable about the community itself, and the factors and forces within it—such as power and politics, legislation and financing, leadership and decision making, health issues and action planning, and, finally, foundations for community change—all of which affect the health of the people in the community.

The WHO Expert Committee has recommended that there be a change in the underlying concepts of health care to improve the results of nursing care in the community. The new and revised concepts should be based on:

1. A health system encompassing the total population rather than focusing on limited groups such as hospitalized patients, self-referrals, or other ready utilizers of available services . . .
2. The acceptance of the community itself as the major determinant of health care, its members being stimulated to recognize and express their needs and expectations and to participate actively in the development, implementation, and evaluation of the health service and health education programme.
3. The possibility that community health may be approached other than through an organized health system . . .
4. The development of nursing as a system of care rather than as a specialized occupation . . .

5. The philosophy that people in a community have a potential for continuous individual development and are capable of dealing with most of their own problems if they are given health education and encouraged by example . . .
6. The need to construct nursing education programmes that embrace all aspects of human life (biological, socioeconomic, and cultural) and that are intimately related to community needs and health practice . . .[12]

Robischon, in discussing community health nursing in a changing climate, has stated:

> We must change our methods and aim our health teaching at populations, rather than individuals. The community nurse of the future, if she is to be skilled as a change agent in promoting health, will need more knowledge about sociocultural patterns, what purposes they serve, how they persist, and how they change. She will also need better understanding of theories of group dynamics, learning, and motivation.[13]

The nature of nursing is derived from the health problems of people. Health, however, must be looked at in the total context of the family and the community. The place of health on the hierarchic scale of values will differ in each community. For example, food has the highest priority for those who are hungry. The fact that communities differ makes it all the more imperative for us to know more about how individual communities view health and change, and why they fail to utilize more effectively many of the services and personnel now available to them. How people try to meet their health problems, where they go when they are in trouble, and whether they reject or accept help are things that the nurse must know in order to work effectively. The nurse must know the factors within a community that enhance the health of the people and those that predispose to poor health; identify the families and groups who are at high risk in relation to health; know the available facilities and their patterns of use or non-use; and guide and support the people in the solution of their own health problems. She must recognize, also, her need to become knowledgeable about such factors and forces within the community itself as power and politics, legislation and financing, leadership and decision making, health issues and action planning, and finally, community change—all of which affect health and health planning. The sphere of action for community health nursing must be the broader community itself, rather than the program of any one specific agency.

The community is where the action is in relation to innovative and evolving health programs and services. It is where community health problems are identified and where significant programs of health promotion and disease prevention, as well as control of major health problems, must be carried out. The community, itself in the process of change, is also the most effective place in which it is possible to bring about improvement in the health status of the people.

One feature of nurse practitioner roles at the present stage of development is the practitioner's competence in physical assessment and health-history taking, in addition to other skills. We believe a similar kind of assessment skill is necessary for what Skrovan, Anderson, and Gottschalk[14] call the community health practitioner. Her skill is in the assessment of the health problems of a community and in mobilizing the people to solve their own health problems. It must be kept in mind that this is not a new venture for community health nursing. However, in this period of rapid increase of new knowledge and new horizons in science and technology, it is imperative that the current practices be congruent with the needs of society.

Community health nursing is changing. It is developing innovative approaches in providing health services, is focusing more and more on the needs of the community rather than the agency, and is collaborating increasingly with many other concerned workers in planning for the community's health. In this period of specialization, fragmentation, and change, community health nursing is a sustaining force and has a vital role to play in furthering and fostering the health of the community. Community health nursing can make its contribution by identifying factors related to health maintenance, prevention of disease, and promotion of health; identifying and interpreting nursing needs in their relationship to broader community health needs; and planning with others for solutions. Community health nursing's specific concern with health may be its point of entry for becoming involved with others in helping to solve some of the broader social problems of the times.

The next four chapters are devoted to exploration of the process by which community health nursing works with the community as the patient.

REFERENCES

1. J. Hanlon, *Public Health Administration and Practice,* 6th edition (St. Louis: C.V. Mosby Company, 1974), p. 314.
2. J. Gardner, "Gardner Hews Out the Great Society," *Newsweek,* February 28, 1966, p. 30.
3. I.T. Sanders, "Public Health in the Community," In H.E. Freeman, S. Levine and L. Reeder, (eds), *Handbook of Medical Sociology* (Englewood Cliffs N.J.: Prentice-Hall, 1965), p. 369.
4. *Ibid.,* p.375.

5. B.F. Mattison, "Community Health Planning and the Health Professions:, *Amer. Jr. Public Health* 58 (June 1968): 1019.
6. D.C. Klein, "The Meaning of Community in a Preventive Mental Health Program," *Amer. Jr. Public Health* 59 (November 1969): 2005.
7. J.W. Alexander, *The Economic Life of Oshkosh* (Madison: University of Wisconsin, Bureau of Community Development, vol. 5, nos. 1 and 2, 1955), pp. 23–24.
8. Klein, op. cit., p. 2005.
9. R. L. Warren, *The Community in America,* 2nd ed. (New York: Rand McNally Company, 1973), p. 9.
10. *Ibid.*, pp. 9–11.
11. WHO Expert Committee, *Community Health Nursing* (Geneva: World Health Organization, Technical Report Series no. 558, 1974), pp. 5, 23.
12. *Ibid.*, pp. 16–17.
13. P. Robischon, "Community Nursing in a Changing Climate," *Nursing Outlook* 19 (June 1971): 413.
14. C. Skrovan, E. Anderson, J. Gottschalk, "Community Nurse Practitioner: An Emerging Role," *Amer. Jr. Public Health* 64 (September 1974): 847–53.

BIBLIOGRAPHY

Alexander, J. W. *The Economic Life of Oshkosh.* Madison: University of Wisconsin, Bureau of Community Development, vol. 5, nos. 1 and 2, 1955.

Conant, R. W. *The Politics of Community Health.* Report of the Community Action Studies Project. Washington, D.C.: Public Affairs Press, 1968.

Freeman, H. E., Levine, S., and Reeder, L. G., eds. *Handbook of Medical Sociology.* Englewood Cliffs, N.J.: Prentice-Hall, 1963.

Gardner, J. "Gardner Hews Out the Great Society." *Newsweek,* February 28, 1966.

Hanlon, J. *Public Health Administration and Practice.* 6th ed. St. Louis: C. V. Mosby Company, 1974.

Hilleboe, H. E. Editorial. "Concepts of Comprehensive Health Planning." *Amer. J. Public Health* 58 (June 1968):1001–2.

———Public health in the United States in the 1970's." *Amer. J. Public Health* 58 (September 1968):1588–1610.

Hitchcock, J. "Working in a Nonhealth Oriented Setting." In *The Nursing Clinics of North America.* vol. 5. Philadelphia: W. B. Saunders Company, 1970, pp. 251–59.

Klein, D.C. *Community Dynamics and Mental Health.* New York: John Wiley & Sons, 1968.

———."The Meaning of Community in a Preventive Mental Health Program." *Amer. J. Public Health* 59 (November 1969):2005–12.

Knight, J. H. "Applying Nursing Process in the Community." *Nursing Outlook* 22 (November 1974):708–11.

Lewis, C. E. "The Thermodynamics of Regional Planning." *Amer. J. Public Health* 59 (May 1969):773–77.

Mattison, B. F. "Community Health Planning and the Health Professions." *Amer. J. Public Health* 58 (June 1968):1015–21.

McGavran, E. G. "Scientific Diagnosis and Treatment of the Community as a Patient." *J. Amer. Med. Assoc.* 162 (1956):723–27.

Mechanic, D. "Ideology, Medical Technology and Health Care Organization in Modern Nations." *Amer. J. Public Health*·65 (March 1975):241–47.

Mott, B. J. "The Myth of Planning Without Politics. *Amer. J. Public Health* 59 (May 1969):797–803.

Olendzki, M. "What Is Community Medicine?" *J. Nurs. Admin.* 2 (September-October 1972):78–86.

Robischon, P. "Community Nursing in a Changing Climate." *Nursing Outlook* 19 (June 1971):410–13.

Sanders, I. *The Community.* 3d ed. New York: Roland Press, 1974.

Sheahan, M. W. "Through Community Action: A Health Commission Reports." *Amer. J. Nurs.* 66 (June 1966):1298–1302.

Skrovan, C., Anderson, W., and Gottschalk, J. "Community Nurse Practitioner: An Emerging Role." *Amer. J. Public Health* 64 (September 1974):847–53.

Smolensky, J., and Haar, F. *Principles of Community Health.* Philadelphia: W. B. Saunders Company, 1961.

Warren, R. E. *The Community in America.* 2d ed. New York: Rand McNally & Company, 1973.

WHO Expert Committee. *Community Health Nursing.* Geneva: World Health Organization, Technical Report Series no. 558, 1974.

CHAPTER 11

GATHERING PERTINENT DATA ABOUT THE COMMUNITY

Community health nurses have a great deal of knowledge about their communities. They serve the families who are the community, and interact with many individuals, groups, and organizations in their behalf. They know the people, neighborhoods, streets, and resources. They participate on innumerable committees, both as professional nurses and as citizens. They have access to records, studies, annual reports, and statistics. They talk to people about the community, read about it, observe it, spend a good deal of their time in it, and obviously have a storehouse of valuable information. Too often, unfortunately, this wealth of knowledge is neither reported, assembled, nor documented. Too often it is hidden away in different and widely scattered files, with the result that when one tries to assess the needs of a community, information which could be most valuable is not available, and important decisions are often made on the basis of inadequate data. These data which have been assembled must be ordered and organized in such a way as to be useful for analysis.

Before any data can be collected, the purpose for which they are to be used must be ascertained. For example, if they are to be used in determining the health problems and nursing needs of a community, the data base may be quite comprehensive. If, on the other hand, they are being applied to the health problems of a specific age group, or of one disease category, the data base should include information that will give clues about these groups. Therefore, it is important to decide in the very beginning what kind of data are needed and for what purpose. The powerful and frequent urge to collect data because it is "interesting" is a serious pitfall and should be avoided.

There is no general agreement about the kind and amount of information that is specific for the determination of the health problems of a community. However, the authors* believe that there are certain kinds of information about a community which provide an overall picture, and serve as a framework for the identification of the health problems from which nursing needs are determined. These kinds of information include:

1. data about the community itself—its physical characteristics and uniqueness
2. information about the people—their distribution and characteristics
3. knowledge about the environment—the housing, air and water, safety, and health-related factors
4. knowledge about the channels of communication, both formal and informal, and the key communicators within the community
5. vital statistics and information about the population—its health and illness patterns and problems
6. data about the health and health-related facilities, resources, and personnel
7. knowledge about available community health nursing services and programs—their resources and interrelationships

Like the information collected for the purpose of working with the family, these kinds of information are important to other health workers as well as to community health nurses. Each discipline, however, will interpret the data in light of its own frame of reference and knowledge. The kinds of questions each profession asks about similar data is an indication of the uniqueness of that health profession to the solution of health problems.

Some of the data outlined above are already available in the community and are readily accessible. For example, related studies may have been done recently in the community. Vital statistics compiled in the health department are usually fairly easy to assemble. The continuing National Health Survey provides information regarding national health problems, though it is difficult, if not impossible, to relate these data to local areas. (One of the aspects of the National Health Planning and Resources Development Act of 1974 is to provide more adequate health data which can be utilized more effectively on a regional or local level.)

The next step is to determine where and how the remaining data can be collected—for example, results of interviews, study of records, comparison of statistics, analysis of ongoing agency programs, and so forth.

*See Appendix B of this text.

Finally, it must be determined who will collect what kind of data. The people in the community who will be most affected by the data, its analysis, and the resulting plan of action should be involved in this very early stage. Many persons in the community can do some of the data collection, will know the key leaders, and are invaluable in keeping the community informed about any progress that is being made. It is also important to get the people involved early, because they are the ones who are going to have major responsibility for carrying out any plans that evolve. The process of gathering pertinent basic data about a community and its people remains the same whether the community is a county, a city, a census tract, the area covered by a nursing organization, or the district of an individual community health nurse.

DATA ABOUT THE COMMUNITY

How can a particular community best be described? What are the unique characteristics that differentiate it from any other community? Is it an inner-city area or neighborhood of a large urban complex? Is it a middle-class suburb with its own form of town government, or a farming community in the South or Midwest? What about its location, climate, and topography—factors which directly influence both the health needs and the patterns of delivery of health services. What are the specific geographic limits of the community? These need to be defined and described as clearly as possible. Parameters may often be delineated by natural boundaries such as rivers and mountains, as well as by roads, streets, or census tracts. The use of census tracts as boundaries fits in with the political jurisdiction. There is less chance of duplication, gaps, and overlapping of statistics when census tracts are used. Census tracts were initially small areas in a community averaging about 4,000 inhabitants, but they are now much larger. The boundaries are usually established jointly by local committees and the Bureau of the Census to achieve some homogeneity of such population characteristics as economic status and living conditions.

Information about the existing form of government is essential for health workers. The health of the community is the legal responsibility of the governmental agency—the health department. The more health workers know about the government and how it affects health, the better able they will be to understand and contribute to the solution of health problems. They must be knowledgeable about such things as how tax money is appropriated for health, and the steps necessary for submitting new legislation and/or supporting or opposing pending legislation. The federal government has become more and more responsive to the health needs of the nation, and the flow of legislation affecting health continues to increase. This makes paramount an understanding of the relationship of local governing groups to those at the state and federal levels.

A brief history of the community is invaluable in these days of regionalization, mobility of industry, city planning, and major highway construction. The problems encountered by a community involved in any one of these major processes are manifold and disruptive and demand considerable community adjustment and change, for no group or community can adjust too far in any direction without upsetting its equilibrium. If change comes about too rapidly, communities are faced at every turn with completely new situations for which they are unprepared.

It is the responsibility of community health nursing, together with other key community workers and institutions, to help a community maintain its equilibrium. Therefore, when major community change is anticipated—change which may be catastrophic to one community yet easily assimilated by another—potential problems must be anticipated. Plans for orientation to and preparation for change must be worked out in advance. Thus, knowledge of what has happened to a community in the past, and of possible plans for the future give perspective to the present and make possible advance planning. The present always lies between the past and the future and must be viewed in this context.

INFORMATION ABOUT THE PEOPLE

Certain kinds of data about the population of community, such as age and sex distribution, ethnic and religious composition, education, and socioeconomic status, should be assembled and considered before any serious assessment of health or nursing needs is attempted.

Change in the total population over the past ten years will give clues about any shift in potential health problems. What is the population per square mile? How is this population distributed spatially? Is it characterized by areas of density and areas of sparseness? These kinds of information are extremely important when one is considering the location, distribution, and delivery of health services. They give clues about some of the health problems which might present.

Knowledge about the percentage of people within each age category contributes to the identification of health needs. What is the proportion of preschool children in relation to the total population? What particular kinds of health services do preschoolers need? Are these currently available? What proportion of community nursing services is directed toward this particular group? Pertinent questions such as these should be asked in relation to each age group within the population.

How many people within the community are 65 years of age and over? This information is important when one is planning for an aging population. The fact that the population is aging has a direct effect upon the whole health picture. In any community with a growing percentage of older people, particular consideration must be given to the gamut of services for prevention and care, the resources for hospital or extended home care, and the supply of supporting personnel so often required by the elderly.

Systematic compilation of information about age and sex of the population does not assure answers about specific health problems. It does, however, give important clues to possible nursing needs and provides a framework of information within which health problems of specific age groups can be studied and looked at in relation to current programs. Many times, studying the age distribution of a population over a period of time brings to light the fact that there has been a population shift. Accompanying changes in priorities of community nursing services should reflect this shift.

The relationship between the health of a community and a variety of its population characteristics—ethnic, socioeconomic, educational, and religious—is well established. These characteristics are as important as age and sex distribution. It is undisputed that health problems are associated with poverty areas, particularly ghettos, with concentrations of socioeconomically and educationally deprived people. Poverty, while not limited to any one ethnic group, is a widespread condition in many groups, such as American Indians, Puerto Ricans, migrants, and blacks. Population characteristics and distribution give valuable clues about the health problems of specific groups, and contribute another dimension to the overall assessment of a community. Comparison of the data about income, occupation, and rate of unemployment with data on financial, educational, vocational, and ethnic distribution will help to pinpoint potential health problems.

KNOWLEDGE ABOUT THE ENVIRONMENT

The American people have finally awakened, and none too soon, to the sorry plight of their environment, and to the havoc wrought by the accelerating technologic development of the last 150 years—technologic development paralleled by increasing pollution of air, water, and land. The frightening spectre of a rapidly diminishing system of life support on earth is before us. Man's future survival may depend upon his understanding and appreciation of the relationship of organisms (man included) to their environment. Community health nurses, as citizens as well as health workers, must be concerned with the environment of the community.

Housing is more than a roof over one's head. It provides the primary environment for children's growth and development, and for family interaction and relationships. It has a great deal to do with the quality of health and of life. The relationship of inadequate and overcrowded habitation to increased health problems—physical, social and emotional—has been well documented. Information about the adequacy of living and housing conditions of the families in the community, about safety, overcrowding, sanitation, insect and rodent infestation, and general state of repair of the houses is basic to any study of health problems. Many of the causes of the current housing crisis are due to the fact that there has been failure to enact and enforce many of the housing codes, regulations, and zoning laws which already exist. There has also been lack of foresight in planning for future housing. Additional information about existing housing regulations and the mechanisms for their enforcement should be sought.

The majority of people take for granted a safe, clean, adequate water supply and do not become unduly concerned until there is a drought or some kind of disaster which makes starkly evident the fact that water is a necessity of the highest priority. The supply of water and the regulations for its safety vary, depending upon the type of community. In a rural farming area which uses well water, for example, the problems related to a safe water supply are different from those of an urban community with a municipal water supply. Knowledge about fluoridation will give clues about the dental health problems which might be found in a community.

A workable plan for garbage, trash, and sewage disposal is mandatory for maintenance of human and environmental health. However, because of the mass of disposable and nondestructible material resulting from our way of life, such a plan is difficult to develop. As with water, waste disposal problems in urban and rural communities may differ strikingly. The concern of a rural community may be a smoking, stinking, rat-infested dump or an overflowing cesspool; while that of an urban area may be trash-littered streets, overturned garbage cans, or overflowing toilets. Sanitary regulations and collection schedules exist in almost every section of the country. Information about the rules, regulations, and standards regarding garbage collection and disposal—and, most important, mechanisms for their enforcement—contributes to the definition of health problems.

Never before in our memory have protective services such as police, fire, and civil defense been so vital. The ongoing responsibilities of maintaining law, order, safety, and protection have been compounded with additional problems associated with an increased crime rate, racial tensions, demonstrations, drug addiction, and violence. In addition to traditional protective services, other resources and programs are often available to a community. They include such things as: transportation services to hospitals and clinics; emergency ambulance services; respirator services; and even educational programs on such topics as alcoholism, drug addiction, and safety. This kind of information is particularly helpful in planning to meet the nursing needs of the community.

Although transportation patterns and resources vary from community to community, particularly between urban, suburban, and rural areas, there is a direct relationship between the availability of transportation and the utilization and delivery of health services. The elderly, the ill, the mother with several small children, the poor, the poorly motivated—these and others are less apt to get to medical facilities if transportation is unavailable, inconvenient, time consuming, or expensive. Lack of parking facilities presents similar difficulties for those with automobiles. Knowledge about transportation routes, frequency of service, costs, transfers, and the transportation problems of any particular segment of the population is essential. In addition, information about planned future changes in transportation patterns, routes, or resources has implications for health planning and may affect decisions about the establishment and location of clinics and other health facilities.

CHANNELS OF COMMUNICATION

Communication, a process by which people exchange ideas and interact, is basic to community life. Within every community there are well-defined formal and informal systems of communication. Informal methods are numerous and tend to operate wherever groups of people collect, such as in hospitals, factories, universities, or wherever conversation is free and easy among people—at the gas station, beauty parlor, or chain store; over the bridge table; or at a neighborhood well-child conference. There are key people within every community who, because of their status or community orientation, are more apt to be an integral part of informal communication which transmits information about local affairs. Without this understanding, one can never hope to develop meaningful, realistic programs. These key people, or high communicators, should be identified. They can be of great help to health workers and should be involved, whenever feasible, in any community health study. Other questions one might ask are: How are decisions made in a particular community? Who makes or vetoes them? Is there a group of decision makers, or do one or two individuals have the final authority?

Formal channels of communication through traditional media such as newspapers, television, radio, telephone, and postal systems are equally important to community life. The press, which includes newspapers, special-interest publications, magazines, and community papers, continues to be a powerful means of community information, ideas, and attitudes. Television, now found in the majority of American homes, is also of significance. Studies and spot checks of television viewers indicate which segment of the population is most likely to be reached at what time of day and on what days. Such information is valuable to community workers for scheduling spot announcements in support of local projects or for dissemination of health information. Knowledge about these existing formal and informal channels of communication is essential to better understand the ways in which ideas, attitudes, and knowledge about health are disseminated, and also how they may be used most effectively for health education.

HEALTH AND ILLNESS PATTERNS

The statistics on a community provide data about the vital eventsthat occur in the population, such as births, deaths, and occurrence of disease. The necessity for a systematic collection of vital statistics was recognized by the federal government at the beginning of the century with the establishment of the Death Registration Area in 1900 and the Census Bureau in 1902. Data about the vital events in a population are basic to the development and evaluation of any community health program. They are also indispensable in any study of community health problems. The number and rate of live births that occur only provide information about the number of persons who are born during any specific period of time. However, this information is necessary for effective planning of facilities of all kinds, such as hospitals, nursery schools, schools, housing, recreation facilities, and health facilities. The number of deaths and the death rate give a picture of the number of people who have died and the incidence of various causes of death over a specific period of time. Caution should be used in defining health problems in a community on the basis of the number of deaths, however, and these data should be looked at in relation to many other factors.

A comparison of birth and death rates of one community with those of adjoining communities, the state, or the nation as a whole gives clues about some of the health problems in a particular community and ideas about the effectiveness of the existing health programs. For example, if the maternal death rate in one community is higher than that of surrounding communities and the state as a whole, this alerts the community to the fact that a problem exists and warrants further exploration.

HEALTH FACILITIES AND RESOURCES

Health facilities and resources dot our communities like raisins in a fruit cake, but there is real question at this point in time about whether there is an actual health care system in America. A system suggests some overall plan or organization. The existence of two systems, one for the "haves" and one for the "have nots" is probably nearer the truth.

Until recently, marked separation prevailed generally between curative and preventive services, with little reaching out on the part of the hospitals into the community and, likewise, little coordination of preventive and health promotional services with those of the hospital. Fortunately, dissatisfaction on the part of many—rich and poor, black and white, consumer and worker, young and old—about the availability, quality, and fragmentation of health care is resulting in a movement toward more comprehensive health planning. The rate and manner of planning are about as varied as the communities which exist, and no two of these are alike. Rapid changes have resulted in much confusion, proliferation, overlapping, and duplication of services and will, no doubt, continue for some time to come. It would take more than a skilled clairvoyant to predict the kind of system that will eventually emerge. There is a general consensus, however, about the fact that there will be change to a new pattern of organization of health services. Currently, several models for a possible national health plan are being discussed and considered.

In order to get as clear a picture as possible about a community's health facilities and resources, data must be systematically compiled about them and their interrelationships. Data must be gathered about the hospitals, clinics, nursing homes, schools, occupational health programs, comprehensive and neighborhood health centers, health maintenance organizations, prepaid group insurance plans, and other health resources. Kinds of data should include: purposes of programs, types of services, numbers of beds, kinds and numbers of personnel employed, utilization of personnel, and the interrelationships which have developed among these various facilities. What about health-related planning groups within the community—such as health or neighborhood councils, councils of health and social agencies, and concerned citizens' groups? Such groups play a vital role in initiating, supporting, and furthering community health. Other questions that might be asked are: Where do people go when they are sick or in trouble? Do they use appropriate or inappropriate community resources? Do they go the doctor, the druggist, or rely on their neighbors? In the last analysis, it is human resources which make community health a reality. In most communities there are human resources in addition to those persons employed in its health agencies. Often nurses, teachers, educators, doctors, social workers, and sociologists—some active and some retired—live within a community and are intimately concerned with its welfare. Faculty from local or neighboring colleges and universities and consultants from state, federal, and other agencies are all important members of a community's human health resources.

INFORMATION ABOUT EXISTING COMMUNITY NURSING SERVICES

If the community health nursing services in many communities could be pictorially portrayed, they would probably look like an old-fashioned crazy quilt, or a collage made up of light and dark oddly shaped patches. Therefore, data about the kinds and extent of available community health nursing services must be collected before any analysis of their adequacy in relationship to need can be attempted. This process involves the systematic collection of data about existing services or agencies. The agency may be voluntary or official, a comprehensive or neighborhood health center, a school, an occupational health or model cities program, or a proprietory home health agency. The purpose of each agency studied needs to be clearly stated. For example, while a voluntary nursing program exists for the provision of community nursing services and education, an official agency such as a health department has much broader purposes, with nursing only one aspect. On the other hand, a neighborhood health center is generally a comprehensive facility providing or arranging for continuous family-centered, preventive, and curative services under one roof for those members of a defined community.

An official agency derives its legal authority from the power of the state through public health law, while a voluntary agency gets its authority by virtue of state incorporation. Authority for the health of school children, however, varies across the country—resting with either the board of health or the board of education, or coming under joint administration.

In order for an agency to qualify as a certified home health agency under Medicare, certain standards for quality control must be maintained, and the inclusion of at least one secondary service such as physical therapy, occupational therapy, or medical social work is mandatory. Agency certification is important in relation to its program and direction.

In 1966 a joint program of accreditation of community nursing services was established by the National League for Nursing and the American Public Health Association. This was the first time that there had been accreditation of any kind for nursing services. This process of accreditation, which includes self-involvement and self-evaluation on the part of the agency, has stimulated and motivated agencies to improve services. It also has given added protection to society for better quality of care. Knowledge of agency accreditation gives one clues as to the quality of service and agency aspirations.

A table of organization of a community health agency provides the basis for a clearer understanding of the relationship of community health nursing to the agency's total program—particularly in regard to authority, responsibility, and channels of communication.

Administrative patterns within organizations are far from uniform, on either the state or local levels, and must be looked at individually. In general, administrative responsibility in voluntary agencies rests with a lay board of directors which has the responsibility for the appointment of an executive director of nurses. On the other hand, administration of a local official agency generally rests with an appointed or locally elected board of health which in turn appoints the health officer. The employment of all other personnel, including nurses, is customarily the prerogative of the health officer (and his advisory committee) but subject to civil service regulations if these exist. Consumer groups are assuming increasing administrative responsibilities for many of the programs in some of the organizations, such as neighborhood health centers and health maintainance organizations. As previously discussed, administration of school health services varies from health department to department of education to joint administration. Whichever plan prevails, it has a direct effect upon the scope and responsibility of the school health service.

Knowledge of the administrative patterns of an agency, such as the composition of its board and advisory committees, its qualifications and standards for appointment of personnel, its channels of communication and processes for decision making, as well as the relationship of nursing within the structure, is necessary for an understanding of the existing nursing services available to the community.

A job description of the nursing director, including such items as educational qualifications and previous experience, gives important clues to the value placed on professional nursing by the board and community. It also clarifies the relationship of the nursing administrator to the health officer, the board of directors, consumer groups, or other administrative bodies, and her lines of communication within the agency and community.

Every organization responsible for using either private or public sources of income must be accountable for its funds and should have a realistic, up-to-date budget and a sound system of accounting. According to Hanlon:

> A sound system of accounting serves many purposes. It provides a financial record of the activities of an agency, reveals its financial condition at all times, provides very necessary data upon which the departmental administrator may base plans for future action, gives substantive protection in case of questions, and provides the fundamental starting point for audits.[1]

Budget problems of home health agencies are becoming increasingly complex. The expansion of third-party payments, contractual agreements, Medicare, and Medicaid have contributed to the complexity. A great deal can be learned about programs, staffing, services, and priorities within the community by studying the budgets of its community health agencies. Financing of health services gives clues about the value a community places on health and its willingness to support it financially.

Public health nurses were the first professional group to study the cost of a nursing visit. They have developed sound methods of cost accounting, some of which have been adopted by other groups. It is useful to know when an agency's latest cost analysis was done, what method was used, and the charge to the recipients of the service.

The success of any community health nursing program depends upon its personnel—their adequacy, quality, and utilization. Twenty years ago one could quote generally accepted minimal staffing requirements per unit of population for basic health services. This is no longer possible. Patterns for the provision of basic services have changed considerably over the past few years. Nonprofessional and paraprofessional workers, with varying kinds of educational preparation, have joined the community health team. Clinical specialists are becoming more and more involved in the community. Many hospital-based home care programs have become more comprehensive and have extended their services into the community. Finally, the consumer has broadened his health aspirations and is playing a much more vital role in the whole area of community health. The establishment of a ratio of community health nurses per unit of population is no longer feasible.

The task of gathering information about health manpower resources is gaining increasing importance because of the maldistribution of health personnel. Information about the numbers of community health nurses, their educational qualifications and experience, and the other nursing resources available needs to be assembled before any analysis of the nursing needs of a community can even be attempted.

Although knowledge about numbers, kinds, and qualifications of personnel is important, it is of no value unless one looks at the ways in which available personnel are utilized to meet the needs of the community. Study of patterns of utilization gives clues to: priorities of service and rationale for nursing assignments; application of new knowledge and trends which have developed; kinds of coordination with other community services; and finally, ways in which contributions of an expanding community health nursing team are integrated and utilized.

There is a need to collect data about the services offered by the different agencies. Who provides bedside care in the community? What about preventive services and health guidance? Are services available for all age groups and disease categories? How many hours per day are the services available? What percentage of people in the community avail themselves of these services? What kinds of clinics are available, and how are they utilized? How broad are the offerings of the school health program? How is school health coordinated with other nursing programs within the community? What kinds of programs—such as community health centers, neighborhood clinics, home care programs, or prepaid group insurance programs—have developed within the community? What nursing services do they offer, and how do these programs relate to other community nursing services? What about any other community programs in which the nurse is involved?

Finally, what patterns and mechanisms for coordination of community health nursing services and what collaborative arrangements, both formal and informal, have been developed within the community? This information can later be studied, as one might study a sociogram, as part of the analysis of community nursing needs. It is through these kinds of arrangements and community relationships that one attempts to tie the resources together into a fabric of community health nursing services which contributes to continuous comprehensive care—the ultimate goal.

This chapter has been concerned with the kinds of data about a community and its people which must be collected and understood by community health nursing as the basis for the next step in the process—analysis of data and identification of nursing needs.

REFERENCE

1. J. Hanlon, *Principles of Public Health Administration*, 3d ed. (St. Louis: C. V. Mosby Company, 1960), p. 299.

BIBLIOGRAPHY

American Nurses' Association. *Standards of Community Health Nursing Practice.* Kansas City, Mo.: American Nurses' Association, 1973.

Bates, F. "Nursing in a Health Maintenance Organization." *Amer. J. Public Health* 62 (July 1972):991–93.

Bruhn, J. G. "The Role of the Public Health Nurse in a Changing System of Nursing Practice." In Stewart, R., and McGill, C., eds. *Maximizing the Nursing Role in Public Health.* San Antonio: University of Texas School of Nursing, 1973 (mimeo).

Carnegie Commission on Higher Education. *Higher Education and the Nation's Health.* New York: McGraw-Hill Book Company, 1970.

Fonaroff, A. "Identifying and Developing Health Services in a New Town." *Amer. J. Public Health* 60 (May 1970):821–28.

Fox, J., Hall, C., and Elerback, L. *Epidemiology: Man and Disease.* New York: The Macmillan Company, 1970.

Hanlon, J. *Principles of Public Health Administration.* 3d ed. St. Louis: C. V. Mosby Company, 1960.

——. *Public Health Administration and Practice.* 6th edition. St. Louis: C. V. Mosby Co., 1974.

Harrelson, E. F., and Donovan, K. "Consumer Responsibility in a Prepaid Group Health Plan." *Amer. J. Public Health* 65 (October 1975):1077–86.

Kessler, I., and Morton, L., eds. *The Community As An Epidemiologic Laboratory.* Baltimore: Johns Hopkins University Press, 1970.

Klein, D. C. "Assessing Community Characteristics." *Community Mental Health J.* 1 (January 1965):301–8.

McKinlay, J., ed. *Research Methods in Health Care.* New York: Milbank Memorial Fund, 1973.

McNeil, H. "How to Become Involved in Community Planning." *Nursing Outlook* 17 (February 1969):44–47.

Means, R. "Interpreting Statistics: An Art." *Nursing Outlook* 13 (May 1965):34–37.

Milio, N. "A Broad Perspective on Health: A Teaching-Learning Tool." *Nursing Outlook* 24 (March 1976):160–63.

Mushkin, S., ed. *Consumer Incentives for Health Care.* New York: PRODIST, 1974.

National Commission on Community Health Services. *A Self Study Guide for Community Health Action.* Vols. 1 and 2. Washington, D.C.: American Public Health Association, 1968.

________ *Health Is a Community Affair.* Cambridge, Mass.: Harvard University Press, 1967.

Ruybal, S. E., Bauwens, E., and Fasla, M. J. "Community Assessment: An Epidemiologic Approach." *Nursing Outlook* 23 (June 1975):365–68.

Salber, E. *Caring and Curing: Community Participation in Health Services*. New York: Prodist, 1975.

Sanders, I. *The Community*. 3d ed. New York: Roland Press, 1974.

Welch, C. "Health Care Distribution and Third-party Payment for Nurses' Services. *Amer. J. Nurs.* 75 (October 1975):1844–47.

CHAPTER 12

ANALYSIS OF DATA AND IDENTIFICATION OF COMMUNITY NURSING NEEDS

Health is caught in a web of environmental, social, and economic influences. The pathology of poverty, as well as inadequate income, unemployment, disability, and excessive mobility necessitate knowledge of social patterns as well as health data. Because of these interrelationships which affect and are affected by health, it is necessary to have access to broad and basic data about the community, its people, and their health, before any meaningful analysis is possible.

The National Commission on Community Services[1] has recommended criteria which can be used as a yardstick for the overall health services of a community, including its community health nursing services. They provide a frame of reference within which to look at health services, and should be kept in mind during the analysis. These are:

1. *Health services should be comprehensive.* To be comprehensive, as the term implies, they should provide health care for all the people in the community who need it wherever they need it—in hospitals, clinics, outpatient departments, extended-care facilities, in school, in place of work, or in the home.
2. *Health care should be continuous and coordinated.* Health care is defined as encompassing total care of the sick, health guidance, disease prevention and rehabilitation, and care for all age groups. This care may be provided by a great variety of people and institutions, such as private physicians, traditional health care institutions, and official and voluntary community health agencies,

as well as by comprehensive and neighborhood health centers, model cities programs, and a myriad of other ways. Irrespective of who provides this care, it should be available to all the people in the community. It should be focused on the needs of the individual, the family, and the community and be continuous and coordinated.

3. *Health care must be available, accessible, and acceptable.* Care may be available to a community as a whole and valuable to those who can or do avail themselves of it. It is of no value, however, for those to whom it is inaccessible or unacceptable, for a complex variety of limitations or reasons.
4. *Health care requires adequate facilities, personnel, and finances.* No community can provide comprehensive care unless it has an adequate amount of all these resources. Communities need to take a long hard look at the places and people who are providing the services, and at other, often innovative ways in which services can be obtained or provided.

These criteria provide desirable yardsticks against which a community and its health services can be studied. It must always be kept in mind, however, that the data which have been collected about a particular community must be analyzed in the light of that community's unique characteristics and particular health problems and needs. Since the problems of no two communities are alike, solutions must be individually tailored. Nursing needs cannot be determined independently or out of context.

The analysis of the information should rest on the data base under each of the categories as discussed in the preceding chapter. The process in the analysis of the data includes:

1. analyzing the data for the relationship and clues to the health status and health problems of a community
2. identifying the health problems
3. identifying the nursing needs
4. analyzing the relationship of the existing community health nursing services to the identified nursing needs
5. determining the priority of nursing needs

THE COMMUNITY

Descriptive information about the community being studied gives one the "feel" of the community and a frame of reference within which to proceed. For example, just knowing that a community is an urban ghetto area, may, it is true, conjure up a stereotype. However, it also gives one some valid and realistic clues that a possible pathologic, health-related complex may exist. On the other hand, if a community is an upper-middle-class suburb, a whole different set of possibilities presents itself. A community may be vastly different from either of these. It may be a metropolitan census tract, or a sleepy New England village. Descriptive and identifying information about the characteristics of the community, its size, location, topography, climate, and population provides a frame of reference within which the relationships of these data may be studied.

The location of a community has a great deal to do with its health. Two very different communities, one an Appalachian settlement isolated by mountains, poor roads, poverty, and cultural privation; and the other, an affluent middle-class suburb firmly connected to a neighboring city by bands of superhighways, will differ in many ways, such as: relationships with neighboring communities; health and health-related problems; availability, accessibility, and utilization of resources; patterns of transportation; socioeconomic and educational levels; and occupational opportunities. Knowledge of geographic location also tells one something about climate, and immediately suggests differences in general as well as seasonal patterns of living—such as the Deep South in comparison with the Northwest or the New England area.

The relationship between the size, or area, of a community and its population, particularly the location of its population, is also revealing. Clustering of low-socioeconomic-level families within certain census tracts of neighborhoods, for example, predicts constellations of problems and indicates need for a very close scrutiny of the data base and the identification of the areas in which further information is needed.

Analysis of the mobility patterns of the population is basic to planners of health services. Mobility and length of residence are particularly important in relation to other factors, such as socioeconomic, ethnic, occupational, and educational considerations. Data of these kinds give one a better understanding of the dynamics of a community. They also give clues about possible kinds of approaches which might be used most effectively in developing a plan for nursing intervention.

Although a large number of federal agencies conduct and finance health activities, the greatest proportion of health services are still provided by private, voluntary, independent, and often specialized agencies. The boundary between public and private programs is often hazy, and not clearly understood. Therefore, analysis of data about existing governmentally sponsored or funded programs, such as Medicare and Medicaid, helps to clarify parameters, relationships, gaps, duplication, and fragmentation of services.

Many times official health programs are planned without adequate involvement either of consumer or other significant and appropriate health workers, including community health nurses. Often today there is antagonism against the bureaucratic structures of governmental agencies. There is a strong desire by the people for more consumer control and input into the services, facilities, and resources.

It is important to know about the patterns and forms of the local government. This information gives access to the local leadership and clues about the channels and mechanisms which can be used to speak for and/or against pending legislation; and to participate in initiating new and additional legislation.

The concept that the past is significant to both the present and the future, a major theme of this book, is directly applicable to analysis of data about a community. Each community, like each individual and family, adjusts to change in its own way. Understanding how change or crisis has been handled in the past makes future behavior more predictable. One community may still be in a state of shock after having recently been bisected by a superhighway. Another community may be struggling with economic depression and unemployment resulting from a prolonged strike affecting its key industry. An extensive redevelopment program may cause disequilibrium in one community, while another will seemingly "take it in its stride." Analysis of what has happened to a community in the past, when it happened, and how the community was able to cope with change gives important clues about its adjustability and dynamics, and the possible timing for introduction of further change.

As important as analysis of the history of a community is knowledge of future change. This is necessary in relation to the assessment of the strengths and weaknesses, and to the timing of anticipated health planning or intervention.

Through the foregoing analysis of the information about the community—description, location, population, government and legislative process, history, and future plans—the relationships between some items in this category have been discussed, and clues about their meaning in the identification of health problems suggested. Analysis of data about each community will no doubt bring to light the need for further questions to be asked, and additional facts to be gathered. All this will result in new relationships and broader understanding of potential health problems, and of the range of ways through which the people may be helped to deal more effectively with their problems.

The analysis of the characteristics of a community's population, the very people who in aggregate give it life and meaning, is of the greatest importance to community health nurses, and is basic to the determination of health problems and nursing needs. The following population characteristics should be explored: age, sex, race distribution, ethnic group composition, religion, educational levels, and socioeconomic factors.

Population takes on meaning to health workers primarily when it is analyzed in terms of its distribution or component parts. For example, the fact that one section of an urban community being studied has a population of 77,000 is important. Further knowledge that the population has decreased by 11.6 percent over the last 6-year period adds another dimension and suggests that those who could afford to do so have moved to better neighborhoods. A look at some of the socioeconomic, occupational, and ethnic characteristics of the community will help to clarify the reason for this population shift.

Many clues about possible health needs can be gleaned from studying the age distribution of a population. For example, the age distribution of the population of 77,000 previously referred to is as follows:

AGE GROUP	PERCENT OF POPULATION
0–19	36.8
20–34	19.0
35–59	28.0
60–64	4.4
65–69	4.1
70–74	3.4
75+	4.3

Possibilities for analysis of these data are manifold. In addition to looking at the overall age distribution and its meaning, one can also focus on each individual segment of the population and study it more definitively. To illustrate, a further breakdown of the age distribution of the younger segment of this population points out that of the 0–19 age group, 32.7 percent are 0–5 years of age; 26.6 percent, 5–9 years of age; 22.4 percent are 10–14 years of age; and 18.3 percent aged 15–19. This additional information about the population will need to be studied carefully in relation to vital statistics, health data, and needs pertinent to each age group. It should then be looked at in relationship to socioeconomic, environmental, and cultural factors if it is to have meaning and relevance to health workers.

Comparison of the age distribution of one population with that of a neighboring community, the state, or the country as a whole further pinpoints population differences and predictable concerns. Also, a look at shifts in age distributions in relation to services and resources for each age category may be both revealing and disconcerting.

Knowledge of ethnicity, race, and religion of a population becomes particularly meaningful when any ethnic or religious group is concentrated within a community or in a particular neighborhood. The cultural values, mores, and customs, for example, prevalent in a predominantly Chinese, Irish, Puerto Rican, or Jewish neighborhood directly influence the way of life, the view of health and illness, and give some ideas about the kind of health program which will be most effective.

It has been stated repeatedly that better educated people demand a higher level of health. Knowledge of the educational level of a population is necessary if health services and programs are to be derived from its needs and desires, and if they are to be understood and accepted by the people.

There is a positive relationship between education and employment, housing, and socioeconomic level. Analysis of the proportion of families within certain income brackets, and of the median income of families in a community, can be very revealing in relation to a community's economics and employment patterns. Although high unemployment is often related to low educational levels and accompanying problems, there may be other national trends affecting the economy and contributing to unemployment. It is evident that an economically depressed community is not able to pay for quality care even if it can be provided. The economic situation within a community has a great deal to do with the establishment of priority of needs. For an economically depressed community, health may have the lowest priority and employment the highest.

THE ENVIRONMENT

The positive relationship between the environment and physical, social, and emotional health, though eminently clear, is seldom afforded the consideration it deserves. A man is intimately and irrevocably dependent upon his environment. He can neither be separated from it nor viewed apart from it. He responds to it with every one of his senses. The environment encompasses innumerable things, conditions, and situations which make up his very way of life. It is one of the major determinants of health problems of individuals, families, and communities.

Today's literature and other communications media are filled with expressions of concern about the ruthlessness and thoughtlessness with which man is destroying the beauty and usefulness of the land, polluting its rivers and streams, and poisoning the air and the very food he eats. Environmental deterioration, the result of the composite of industrialization and technology, a rapidly expanding population, and a mobile urban society, gives justifiable cause for concern and is particularly significant to health workers.

Several key environmental factors pertinent to health have been selected for analysis. They include housing, air, water, sanitation, safety and protective measures, and, finally, transportation. Community health nursing must be alert to these and any additional environmental factors which potentially might have an adverse effect on health, such as stress factors associated with the environment. Analysis of data about a community in which an airplane factory, for example, is a key industry may suggest clues to possible pollution and other health problems. Further exploration may either prove that there is a health hazard or may give evidence of the fact that adequate and careful health regulations are providing effective controls.

There is a direct relationship between health and housing. Therefore, analysis of data about the availability, adequacy, and acceptability of housing in a community gives clues about possible health hazards as well as socioeconomic status. For example, if analysis indicates that 50 percent of a community's housing is in fair to poor condition, and is occupied predominantly by blacks and Puerto Ricans, one can predict that health and health-related problems will differ from those of a neighboring middle-class suburb. The amount of crime and delinquency will be greater, accidents will be more frequent, and fires will occur more often. It can also be predicted, with certainty, that social and emotional problems associated with overcrowding and confusion will abound, and that infectious diseases, rat bites, and lead poisoning will occur with relatively high frequency. Analysis of these data suggests the need for a variety of protective, educative, and supportive services. It may also reveal such things as landlord exploitation of tenants, unsafe habitation, or failure of enforcement of existing housing codes and regulations. The community health nurse may need to become the advocate of the residents of the community for better living conditions.

Analysis of data concerning water supply, sanitation, sewerage, and trash disposal programs becomes particularly meaningful when viewed in relation to the concentration of population, its housing, and its needs. For example, if a particular housing development is expanding at such a rapid rate that sewerage, trash, garbage collection, and even a safe water supply are inadequate, there is obviously a potentially serious health problem. On the other hand, properly tested well water and cesspools may be perfectly safe and adequate for a rural community.

Protective services such as fire, police, civil defense, and safety must also be viewed in relationship to the population and its whole way of life. For example, in one very old section of a New England city, the streets (actually alleys) proved to be so narrow that it was impossible for fire equipment even to enter some of them. Residents of many of the apartments, which were inadequately heated, used space heaters—a practice which had serious consequences and resulted in devastating fires, burns, and poisoning from ingestion of fumes from kerosene. Fortunately, analysis of these data led health workers and concerned citizens to later select this area for urban redevelopment.

Analysis of the kind and frequency of accidents, assaults, and molestation of the population indicates the importance of gathering further data about such factors as how, where, and when the incidents occurred; what resources and facilities are available for prevention; what more are needed; and what are the best plans for future action.

In Part I of this book transportation was selected as one of the vital forces which contributed to the development of the country. Transportation is equally important to our way of life today. As might be expected, however, many of the current problems associated with it have changed.

Analysis of the kinds of transportation—trolley, bus, train, and automobile—and routes and patterns of transportation within and between communities gives health workers invaluable information about how people can get to shops, to health facilities, homes of other family members, how long travel to desired destinations takes, and how many changes or transfers are necessary; what expense the travel entails; how convenient the transportation is from place of residence to points of destination; and how well schedules are kept. Analysis of these and other pertinent data gives invaluable clues about location of health resources, patterns of utilization of the services, and planning for different types and locations of future facilities. It provides the basis for consideration of the need for alternate kinds or sources of transportation.

The tension, and even damage to hearing, which can be caused by the roar and sonic boom of airplanes or the constant hum of superhighway traffic are often overlooked. Having information about situations of this kind in a community located adjacent to a large metropolitan airport or a superhighway can give some clues about possible physical or emotional problems.

Transportation is vital to our whole way of life. Mounting problems, such as congestion, traffic jams, accidents, and air pollution, all associated with urbanization, and all related to health, are demanding that communities come up with innovative solutions to transportation problems.

In this category, we have looked at some of the environmental factors which interface with other factors in a community, and give clues about possible or potential health problems. It is only when some of the environmental hazards are decreased or eliminated that the health status of the people in a community will improve.

COMMUNICATION

Just as transportation is necessary for the movement of people and goods between and within communities, so is communication vital to man's whole way of relating, learning, teaching, sharing, asking, helping, collaborating, and just living with and trying to understand his fellow man. Technologic and scientific developments have resulted in a proliferation of communications media such as television, radio, tape recorders, and telephones. Amounts and kinds of printed materials have also mushroomed. Analysis of the kinds of media which are available to a community, and how and to what extent they seem to be used, gives health workers clues about how widely the population may have been exposed to health and health-related information in the past. It also gives some ideas about the communication resources appropriate for possible future health education and guidance programs.

Equally important is the analysis of informal sources of communication. Identification of individuals, groups, and organizations that tend to take leadership in either supporting or opposing community changes gives health workers a better understanding of community dynamics. It is important to learn who the real leaders, or "gatekeepers" of information, are in the community. They are the persons who have a large part to play in the development and nurturing of the norms and values held by a community. These persons may not be in the leadership positions, but they may be the first ones to whom the people in a community turn for approval before any changes can be implemented. Community health nurses, because of their close proximity to the people, probably are in a strategic position to know who these "gatekeepers" are. They should be identified very early, as one can never hope to develop meaningful and realistic health programs without their support and involvement.

It is also important to determine what the other channels of communication are. Who talks to whom? For what reasons? Who are the high communicators? What do they communicate? Are they listened to?

In this category, we have discussed the various channels of communication, both formal and informal, in a community. Effective communication is one of the high priorities today. There are even some who think that lack of communication between health professionals and consumers may be the major health problem in the country.

HEALTH AND ILLNESS

Any meaningful health program must be planned in relation to the problems and needs of each community. Health problems cannot be identified until there has been careful analysis of data about the health of the people, the vital statistics, the incidence and prevalence of disease, and the leading causes of death. The unique problems of a particular community, such as one harboring a nuclear power plant or a coal industry, would indicate the need for additional data relative to these characteristics.

Analysis of the vital health statistics of a community parallels the medical history of a patient, or the analysis of the health problems of a family, in terms of its importance in determining a community's health. To illustrate, knowledge that the infant death rate of a community is 30.2 does not really pinpoint the factors which account for this elevated rate. A look at the infant death rate of a community by census tracts, however, gives a much clearer picture. It may reveal that the rates in the two most heavily populated census tracts are 52.4 and 50.6 respectively. Further information may reveal that these are areas characterized by poor housing, considerable unemployment, and a high rate of illegitimacy; and also that two-thirds of the residents are either first- or second-generation foreign born. These kinds of data also give clues about some of the socioeconomic and health-related problems of mothers and children which may exist in the community, and which should be investigated more definitvely. They may indicate the need for special services for pregnant women, for child health supervision, for health guidance, and for services to adolescents. The same "focusing" process used in relation to the infant death rate can be applied to any other data about the community. It might well be used in relation to the maternal mortality rate in helping to determine the major factors which contribute to maternal mortality, and the necessity for improved programs and services.

Analysis of the incidence and prevalence of heart disease, cancer, diabetes, and any other disease significant to a particular community must be carried out in relation to factors such as the age distribution of the population, the socioeconomic status, and available resources. Clues to the health problems and their priorities, which are basic to planning, can then be identified.

Analysis of the leading causes of death can be helpful in a variety of ways. For example, if the leading cause of death in one community is infectious disease, while that of the state or nation is heart disease, there are clear implications for exploring sanitation, the availablilty of preventive health programs, and the adequacy of medical care and hospital facilities. On the other hand, if accidental death occurs frequently, data concerning the kinds and locations of accidents, and the amount of disability that results, should be collected. The community's resources for safety and for the prevention of accidents should also be explored. If one of the leading causes of death (for example, heart disease) is inconsistent with that of the state or the nation, what are the causes of this? What resources and facilities are available for prevention, for care, and for rehabilitation for those with this health problem?

An analysis of the health and illness data for a community gives some clues about the rise and fall in the illness level, birth and deaths, the utilization of health facilities, and the various types of available health personnel. Mattison[2] describes these data as taking the temperature and pulse of a community. Patterns of health and illness in the community over time can also be garnered from these data.

HEALTH FACILITIES AND RESOURCES

Inherent in the concept of comprehensive health care is the adequacy and quality of health resources, facilities, and personnel available. Analysis of information about hospitals, clinics, extended-care facilities, and other health and health-related institutions will give clues about the adequacy and kinds of facilities, as well as their relationships to the health priorities of the people they serve. To illustrate, if in a community the incidence and prevalence of chronic disease is high, evaluation of the kinds of resources which are available to this group is specifically indicated. Analysis of health data about each segment of the population aids in the determination of health problems, their priority, and possible solutions.

Just as vital statistics and health data give life and meaning to the determination of health problems and needs in a community, so do health and health-related personnel give life and meaning to health facilities and resources. The growing army of professionals, professional assistants, specialists, consumers, neighborhood workers, and others has much to contribute to comprehensive care. To do this in any unified way, however, its members will have to learn different ways to communicate, and to coordinate their efforts in order to avoid the fragmentation and confusion which now exist. Analysis of the kinds and numbers of personnel available to a community is necessary, as no health program will succeed without well-prepared personnel in sufficient numbers. Analysis of personnel resources also gives additional clues about how the various health workers might make the best contribution to a community—either by direct service, coordination of services, collaboration with others, or in a consultant capacity.

In this category, the necessity for having knowledge about the availability of health resources and facilities has been highlighted, and some thoughts about how these data can be utilized were shared.

COMMUNITY NURSING SERVICES

There are certain data-base items which nursing must have about the organizations and agencies providing community health nursing services within a particular community. These include the types and extent of services provided; their availability, accessibility, and acceptability; comprehensiveness; utilization; costs; and personnel. Also necessary are the kinds and extent of relationships and the patterns of intercommunication which have been established between the agencies and the personnel providing the services.

Community health nursing services in one community may be provided by a one-nurse agency, and in another by a veritable patchwork of voluntary, official, and specialized agencies. A mass of data about any or all of these programs is meaningless until, as has been pointed out, it is analyzed in relation to the health problems and nursing needs of the people.

First, and extremely important, is consideration of the kinds of community health nursing services available to a community. Is there provision for health maintenance, which includes bedside care of both the acutely and the chronically ill; for rehabilitative nursing; for prevention of disease; and for health promotion? The kinds of services provided may be comprehensive, but are they available for all age groups? For example, a hospital-based home care program may provide a gamut of hospital and home care services to its own patients, but what about others in the community who need nursing services?

If the services are comprehensive and available to all age groups, are they accessible? Are they convenient to public transportation? The relationship between a community's transportation and the location of its health facilities will provide important information in answering questions about utilization of the services. If data indicate that 30 percent of the case load of the neighborhood clinic comes from another area of the city, how are the needs of the rest of the residents being met? What other factors might account for the fact that so few people take advantage of the resources? Is the service acceptable to the people, or are there cultural or financial barriers which prevent maximum utilization? The relationship between utilization of the services and the characteristics of the population will contribute to a further understanding of these questions.

The cost of care is one of the factors which influence patterns of utilization of services. Information about the cost to the agency providing service, as well as the cost to the patient, often points out directions for exploration of other possible sources of financing. The cost to the patient must be analyzed in relationship to available third-party payments, such as Medicare, Medicaid, or the American Cancer Society, as well as to the socioeconomic levels of the community in general.

Analysis of data about the personnel providing community health nursing services gives clues about the possible quantity, quality, and service patterns. If, for example, a large percentage of community health nurses in a particular community are experienced and are educationally prepared; it can be assumed that the potential for quality of service is present. Additional information about such things as supervision, staff development, and team functioning gives further clues about the possible extent and quality of the nursing services offered.

Study of the kinds of referrals and contractual agreements which have been developed among the nursing organizations gives clues about coordination of services and continuity of care. Additional information about community health nursing's participation on community planning groups adds another dimension to one's understanding of nursing's involvement in the community. The referral sources of individuals and families/groups to the community health nursing services provides some clues about the knowledge the community has of the available nursing services. In turn the referral arrangements the community health nursing services have with other health facilities gives some ideas about continuity and comprehensiveness of nursing care. There is renewed discussion today about continuity of care from the hospital to the home and of the vital role nursing has to play in this endeavor. Some state health departments have passed regulations which require that a community health nurse or a social worker be employed to take responsibility for planning for continuity of care before patients are discharged from the hospital.

All of the nursing services in a community must be looked at in order to have a composite picture of the nursing system. The community health nursing leaders should take a leadership role in working with other nursing leaders to make the nursing system responsive to the nursing needs of the community. In doing this the potential nursing's contribution to improvement of the health status of the people will come nearer to fruition.

We have looked at some of the clues to the real and potential health problems under each category. It is now necessary to look at the relation of each of the categories to the other to determine the health problems. What is the relationship, for example, of unemployment to the incidence of alcoholism, suicide, and accidents? What part do the media play in health education of the community, and what might be the possible consequences if some of the information is incorrect or misleading? How does the way of life of the people and their health practices affect their health problems? Health practices such as overeating, lack of exercise, smoking, and social crowding are more important precursors to health problems than available medical technology and treatment facilities. A critical analysis of the items in each of the categories will result in the determination of the health problems. The health problems should be listed in order of priority, with the one with the highest priority at the head of the list.

Throughout we have defined a nursing need as the contribution nursing can make to the solution of a health problem. We have also indicated that some health problems will have more nursing needs than others—and that some health problems may have no nursing needs. In addition, there may be nursing needs which are being met adequately by other health resources in the community. Consequently, those needs will have a low priority for the community health nurse.

When the health problems of a community are chronic disease, infectious disease, or maternal and child health, for example, nursing obviously has an important and vital role to play in meeting the community's nursing needs. The health concern of greatest priority in another community, however, may be about an adequate water supply for an expanding population. This is of concern to community health nurses, but it is of major concern to the sanitary engineer. He is the one the community must turn to for solutions, rather than to nursing. The health problems of yet another community may be drug addiction among teenagers. In this instance, analysis of the number and variety of personnel, in addition to community health nurses, who are currently actively involved in developing a drug program within a community, will help to pinpoint what and how community health nurses might best contribute. It may well be that there are several other high-priority health problems with more pressing nursing needs. Nursing may decide that in this instance it will not become actively involved with the drug problem, but will work with others in a supportive and perhaps consultative role.

In a community in which the majority of the residents are older retired persons, one of the major health problems might well be chronic disease. If analysis of the available community health nursing service to this population indicates that such services as bedside nursing in the home, rehabilitation, and extended-care facilities are not adequately provided, but that the bulk of the nursing services of the community are for mothers and children, then it is evident that the nursing needs of this community are not being met. To illustrate, it is not unusual in a community where the maternal and child needs are the most pressing, that the major emphasis of nursing service tends to be devoted to bedside nursing care of the sick. Further analysis of situations of this kind may well prove that the financial problems of an organization, coupled with the availability of income from federal sources such as Medicare, have influenced the directions in which the programs have developed—and all too often, away from preventive and educative services. It must always be kept in mind that basic preventive and protective programs, such as those for tuberculosis and other communicable diseases, should always be maintained.

In this chapter, we have indicated the steps in the determination of health problems and of nursing needs in a community. Some of the clues which are highlighted by the data base were discussed, and some of the relationships of the data from each category were mentioned. The relationship between the nursing needs of a community and its health problems was discussed, and a determination of the priorities of the nursing needs was explored. This kind of determination helps to keep the nursing needs and goals in focus, and ensures that the contribution and efforts of nursing will be directed toward solutions of the health problems of a community. In the next chapter, the development of a nursing plan of action will be explored.

REFERENCES

1. National Commission on Community Health Services, *Health Is a Community Affair* (Cambridge, Massachusetts: Harvard University Press, 1967).
2. Mattison, B.F. "Community Health Planning and the Health Professions." *Am. J. Public Health 58* (June 1968), p. 1019.

BIBLIOGRAPHY

American Nurses' Association. *Standards for Community Health Nursing Practice.* Kansas City, Mo.: American Nurses' Association, 1973.

Bernal, H. "Power and Interorganizational Health Care Projects." *Nursing Outlook* 24 (July 1976):418–21.

Duhl, L., ed. *The Urban Condition.* New York: Simon and Schuster, 1969.

Fox, J., Hall, C., and Elverback, L. *Epidemiology: Man and Disease.* New York: The Macmillan Company, 1970.

Freeman, R. "Nurse Practitioners in the Community Health Agency." *J. Nurs. Admin.* 4 (December 1974):21–24.

Knight, J. "Applying Nursing Process in the Community." *Nursing Outlook* 22 (November 1974):708–11.

Lindaman, F. and Costs, M. "The Voice of the Community." *Amer. J. Public Health* 62 (September 1972):1246–48.

Mattison, B.F. "Community Health Planning and the Health Professions." *Amer. J. Public Health* 58 (June 1968):1015–1021.

Means, R. "Interpreting Statistics: An Art." *Nursing Outlook* 13 (May 1965):34–37.

National Commission on Community Health Services. *A Self Study Guide for Community Action.* vols. 1 and 2. Washington, D.C.: American Public Health Association, 1968.

———. *Health Is a Community Affair.* Cambridge, Mass.: Harvard University Press, 1967.

Price, J., and Vincent, P. "Program Evaluation: What to Ask before You Start." *Nursing Outlook* 24 (February 1976):84–87.

Richardson, J. D., and Crutchfield, F. D. "Priorities in Health Care: The Consumer's Viewpoint in an Appalachian Community." *Amer. J. Public Health* 63 (February 1973):79–82.

Sparer, G., and Alderman, A. "Data Needs for Planning Neighborhood Health Centers." *Amer. J. Public Health* 61 (April 1971):796–806.

Spradley, B. W. *Contemporary Community Nursing.* Boston: Little, Brown and Company, 1975.

CHAPTER 13

DEVELOPING A NURSING PLAN OF ACTION FOR THE COMMUNITY

The process of planning is given the highest priority today. A new era of planning in America has been brought into sharp focus by many forces operating within an increasingly complex society: a national policy that health is the right of each individual; the active participation of nonprofessionals in an expanding health team; a greater knowledge of the direct relationship between illness and health; a national mandate for comprehensive health planning; a new interest and better technology for early detection of possible ills; an emphasis on the needs of people rather than on agencies; and finally, the realization that only through planning can something be done about the "wonderful and awful" health system which has evolved in America.

Planning is the basis for action, and this is an era of social action, as well as for planning. There is heightened awareness on the part of many who are involved with health that only through the concerted and collaborative efforts of both health professionals and citizens can this country begin to cope with its new and changing health hazards, and to utilize its resources appropriately to meet the present and future health problems.

The National Health Planning and Resources Development Act of 1974 (P.L. 93–164) replaces the earlier legislation relating to comprehensive health planning, regional medical programs, and the construction of health and hospital facilities.

Among the highlights of the Act is a list of national health priorities. This is a "first" for the United States. The health priorities are:

a. The provision of primary care services for medically underserved populations, especially those which are located in rural or economically depressed areas.
b. The development of multi-institutional systems for coordination or consolidation of institutional health services.
c. The development of medical group practices, health maintenance organizations, and other organized systems for provision of health care.
d. The training and increased utilization of physician assistants, especially nurse clinicians.
e. The development of multi-institutional arrangements for the sharing of support services necessary to all health service institutions.
f. The promotion of activities to achieve needed improvements in the quality of health services, including needs identified by the review activities of PSROs [Professional Service Review Organizations].
g. The development of health service institutions of the capacity to provide various levels of care on a geographically integrated basis.
h. The promotion of activities for the prevention of disease, including studies of nutritional and environmental factors affecting health and the provision of preventive health care services.
i. The adoption of uniform cost accounting, simplified reimbursement and utilization reporting systems, and improved management procedures for health service institutions.
j. The development of effective methods of educating the general public concerning proper personal health care and methods for effective use of available health services.

Another "first" is the establishment of a National Council on Health Planning and Development, and the development of national guidelines for health planning.

In addition, the Act provides for establishment of Health Service Areas within each state, for planning and development of health services. Health Systems Agencies (HSAs) are to be established for each of the health service areas. The membership of the HSAs is to include: 60 percent consumers—broadly representative—no one who has been a provider of health care within 12 months of appointment; health care providers; health care institutions; health care insurers; health professional schools; and allied health professionals. Not more than one-third of the membership are to be health providers. Other features of the Act include State Health Planning and Development Agencies, State Health Coordination Councils, a State Medical Facilities Plan, and Regional Centers for Health Planning.[1]

The implications of this Act are not known at this time. However, the potential for the improvement of the health status of the people as a whole is implicit. Only implementation of the features of the Act will determine how well the potentials will be realized.

Community health nurses from the beginning worked with people in the community and were concerned with their health. Today, community health nurses are part of a multifaceted health complex and are functioning in new roles in this expanding system. Their responsibility is greater than ever. They must take leadership in identifying health problems and nursing needs, and in mobilizing people to solve their own health problems. They are also participating in the planning and decision-making process, and in finding innovative ways to provide nursing services and developing mechanisms by which these services will reach those who need them—the consumers.

There are forces within community health nursing itself which make planning urgent: changing patterns for financing nursing care resulting from legislation such as Medicare; changing roles and responsibilities resulting from multipurpose patterns of nursing education and the expanding role of the nurse; proliferating health services, which include community health nursing; increasingly complex nursing care provided in the home; priority of comprehensiveness; pressure from the consumer for better health care; proprietary home health agencies; need for availability of services over a 24 hour period; shorter hospitalizations; Professional Service Review Organizations (PSROs); renewed emphasis on accountability; and P.L. 93-164.

Who should take the initiative in determining that something should be done about a community nursing need, for discussing it with concerned others, and for helping to turn the wheels for action? More specifically, who is responsible for initiating community health nursing planning? It is clearly the responsibility of the community health nurse, since the community is her patient. However, she has not always assumed leadership but has all too often sat back and waited for someone else to take the intiative. Too often the needs of an agency or a particular geographic area have been the focus for action. Too often nurses in key positions within the community have exerted influence in relation to their own agency's program and vested interest, without necessarily taking into consideration the nursing needs of the broader community. This does not suggest that the total responsibility for planning community health nursing rests with nursing alone. The task of planning is too important and too big to leave entirely to nurses. It also demands the best thinking, resources, and skills of many others. Nursing, however, has primary responsibility for seeing that the nursing needs of the community are met. It must determine what it can do best, and when it needs to call on others for assistance and guidance.

For purposes of clarification, the process of developing a plan of action to meet the nursing needs of the community is presented here as a series of separate and consecutive steps. This is done with full realization that there is some danger in this segmental approach, since in reality the steps are interrelated and often interchangeable. These steps are:

1. Preplanning to meet the identified nursing needs.
2. Exploring factors to be considered in establishing the nursing plan of action.
3. Determining the long-term and short-term nursing goals.
4. Evaluating the alternative actions for reaching the nursing goals.
5. Selecting the action to reach the nursing goals.

PREPLANNING TO MEET THE IDENTIFIED NURSING NEEDS

Preplanning provides opportunity for decision making about who should be involved in the planning, and for the determination of the parameters or limits within which a plan is to be developed. In other words, some preliminary decisions are made at this time, and the stage is set for developing an effective nursing plan.

Who should be involved in developing the nursing plan? Should community health nurses do this alone, or should it be done in conjunction with others? The nature and extent of the nursing needs, and the size and complexity of the community and its health problems, will help to determine who should be involved. Consideration should be given to:

1. Those for whom the plan is designed—the consumers. The consumer, like the community health nurse, has his area of expertise. He is the one who can best interpret the desires, interests, and needs of the people. The final decision about any plan of action rests with him.
2. Those who are concerned with the health problems. Professionals and other health-related groups who are concerned with the effect of the health problems on the community should be involved in the formulation of the plan of action.
3. Those who appear best able to contribute to the plan by virtue of their ability, position, knowledge, or experience.
4. Those persons who are most likely to follow through in carrying out the plan of action because of interest, power, motivation, or professional skills.

Many other members of the health team and the community, as well as nurses, have a vital stake in health and a valuable contribution to make to the solution of community health problems. The primary responsibility of nursing, however, still rests with nursing—just as the ultimate success of community action rests with the citizen for whom it is undertaken.

Any planning group, no matter how well selected or representative, can be so large that it becomes unwieldy and unproductive. Everyone concerned with the problem cannot personally be represented in its alleviation, but the interests of those who are concerned can and must be considered in the deliberations. This can be done by the inclusion of representatives who are acceptable to those whom they represent, and who are qualified to speak for them. Others can be added or consulted whenever this seems desirable. It may be necessary to hold several preliminary discussions with key persons before deciding who will become directly involved in the development of the plan of action.

FACTORS TO BE CONSIDERED IN ESTABLISHING THE NURSING PLAN OF ACTION

Inherent in this step of the planning process is recognition that there are many factors operating within a community which can influence the plan either positively or negatively. Some of the factors which may affect the success or failure of a plan are: possible barriers to community change, such as vested interests, traditions, patterns of organization, and finances; forces within the community such as politics and power; factors such as previous experience and timing; and contemporary concepts related to planning, such as community of solution and regionalization.

It is one thing to spell out the steps in planning for community health nursing, and another to carry them out in today's complex, changing, and, to date, unclear situation. One is tempted to look back on the pattern of yesterday's community health nursing service with a certain nostalgia. It seems to have been so simple. Most public health nursing services were provided by either the official or voluntary nursing program. In reality it was almost monopolistic. Basic responsibilities were spelled out for the official agency. The voluntary nursing agencies, for the most part, decided what services they would provide, determined their costs, and decided whom they would employ. Exclusive of those public health nursing programs which were generalized or combined, lines of demarcation between the official and voluntary programs were quite clearly understood. Although it would be presumptuous to claim that those traditional services were consistently of the best quality, or inclusive, there was in most communities a recognizable, discernible network of community health nursing services. There is little relationship between the situation of yesterday and that of today in most communities, particularly in metropolitan areas. New and different services, both comprehensive and specialized, are provided by satellite clinics, neighborhood centers, and home care programs, to name a few. Some of these have carved out islands of special services for selected groups and have left gaps and holes in a former, though perhaps thin, community nursing fabric. The agencies which traditionally provided most of these services have adjusted to the changes in a variety of ways. In some instances they have taken leadership in the development of innovative programs. In others, through contractual agreements, they have provided staff or services to a variety of programs. It must be recognized that the health market today is competitive in terms of patterns of service and organization, as well as manpower. There is also competition in relation to finances. Revenue from United Funds, traditionally an important source of income for many voluntary nursing agencies, is less abundant today. Increasingly, a larger proportion of this source of income is directed toward the needs of inner cities. This trend is of grave concern to suburban communities and is causing them real financial problems and worries. It is true that there are additional sources of income through federal programs such as Medicare and Medicaid, which pay for a growing amount of care. Federal financing, however, influences the direction and emphasis of the programs which provide these kinds of care. It must be recognized that there are almost as many vested interests as there are programs providing community health nursing services, and at present there is very little agreement about just what the most desirable pattern for the future ought to be. All these factors influence and affect any planning relative to community health nursing. Any planning group, no matter how representative, will need to come to grips with the relationship between these vested interests and what is best ultimately for the greatest number of people within the community—for the consumer and not the agency. Therefore, vested interests and traditions, as well as patterns of organization and financing, can be barriers to change and can influence planning.

There are other factors which must be taken into consideration in developing a nursing plan of action for the community. One of these is politics—politics in the sense of how a group arrives at what is best for it, its goals. This kind of politics includes the efforts of the planners, as individuals and respresentatives of organizations, to utilize their skill, power, and persuasiveness to obtain their desired goals. This takes not only leadership but also cooperation and willingness to arbitrate. It also demands flexibility and real interest in a common goal.

Closely allied to politics is power. Milio[2] describes organizational effectiveness as the capacity of an organization to bargain for scarce resources. Whoever has the most power gets the resources. Every system within a community has its power structure, and community health nursing is no exception. The larger, or richer, or more prestigious community health nursing agencies have usually had the most power in decision making, and have often used this in the community through informal decisions made by relatively few people. Prestige is power and so is money. The source of a great deal of new money for community health nursing services today is the federal government. The federal government is big power, but the federal system at the present time is not designed for partnership. The extent to which community health nursing programs within a community are dependent upon federal funds and regulations is a factor of growing importance today and one which must be reckoned with in developing any nursing plan. In the end, each community must work out its own community health nursing program to fit its own politics and power, its own special problems and resources, and its own community personality.

Community health nurses must carefully consider the timing for any plan of action. Timing may be the key factor in the success or failure of any plan. Improper timing may result in apathy or strong resistance to any suggestion, resistance due in reality to factors unrelated to community health nursing. For example, the community may have just been through a period of rapid change and upheaval by virtue of a massive redevelopment program. It may need to regain its equilibrium before tackling further problems. Conversely, acceptance of a plan may be made easier because a particular community is interested in and ready for change and accepts social action and progress as valuable. The priority which the community places on a particular problem at a particular time is part of the picture. Sensitivity to the pulse of the community, therefore, is of the essence in developing the nursing plan of action. Closely related to timing are the past experiences of a community and the ways in which it has previously responded to change. Also important are the composition of the community, the extent of involvement of its citizens in community affairs, and the relationships which have been developed.

It must always be kept in mind that any community, big or small, is part of a larger society and must be looked at within this context. The ways in which contemporary society views health problems, and the kinds of approaches it is using for their solution have a real impact on a community plan for nursing. There are two concepts in particular which should be considered. They are "community of solution" and "regionalization."

As previously pointed out, no individual community can or necessarily should provide all its own health services, resources, or facilities. It cannot, likewise, find solutions for all the problems within its own boundaries. The National Commission on Community Health Services suggests:

> that where health services are concerned the boundaries of each community are established by the boundaries within which a problem can be defined, dealt with, and solved.[3]

And further that:

> As the center of responsibility for assuring that personal and environmental health services are available to all residents, the community should first assay its resources, its programs and needs, and the strengths that exist to meet these needs. After the community has assessed its resources, it can join with other communities to solve larger problems that require resources of a larger geographic region, a wider political jurisdiction, and more funding than is available to one locality.[4]

This concept of the community of solution is of the utmost importance to community health nurses in the plan which ensues. The needs of a mobile population are constantly changing, and each new problem must be studied in relation to the particular boundaries within which it can be solved. For example, a community's need for home health services may be far better met by arrangements through a contractual agreement to purchase these from a large, well-established agency in a neighboring community, rather than establishing its own. This concept can also be applied to better utilization of the larger health team.

Closely related to the concept of community of solution is that of regionalization. Although each community is unique, adjoining communities or areas have many common interests, as well as problems. It is reasonable that planning for health services within geographic regions having similar interests and problems makes possible better use and distribution of resources, facilities, and money. The federal government gave little direct encouragement to regional planning for health until 1966 when the 89th Congress passed the Regional Medical Programs Act and the Comprehensive Health Planning Act. Inherent in the Health Resources and Development Act of 1974 is the solving of health problems on the basis of community of solution and/or regionalization of service.

There is heightened interest in regionalization of nursing services and the utilization of this concept in planning. Many community health nurses, as well as other health workers, know that regionalization of health services is paramount and will come about some day. Questions and fears are being raised about who will control these regional community health nursing services, who will be left out, and what the implication will be for official and voluntary nursing services alike.

There may be one goal or several goals toward which action is to be directed. For example, let us assume that the health problem of the highest priority in one particular community, determined on the basis of all the data, was found to be in the maternal and child care area; that nursing services, resources, and facilities for mothers and children were also inadequate; and that a whole constellation of nursing needs was identified. In such a situation the specificity and clarity with which community health nurses state their desired goals for mothers and children can make a great deal of difference to planning. Too often the goal is stated as "provide comprehensive health care for mothers and children." One cannot deny that this is an exemplary statement. It would be just as heretical to be against comprehensive care as against motherhood itself, but it is, like the pot of gold at the end of the rainbow, hard to reach. The fact is that such an abstract, nonspecific, all-inclusive goal does little to point out to those attempting to attain it the best road for them to follow. Equally important, how can one measure or evaluate specific progress toward such a diffuse goal? The point to be made here is that goals need to be stated in clear, measurable, behavioral terms which in turn can serve as measuring rods for progress toward attainment. Community health nurses, therefore, should carefully determine what they expect the outcomes to be in meeting the nursing needs of mothers and children in the community. Some of the long-term goals might be stated as follows:

1. All high-risk pregnant women will receive nursing supervision within 18 months.
2. Private physicians and clinics providing maternity services will refer all high-risk pregnant women for nursing supervision within three years.
3. All premature infants will receive home nursing supervision within one year.
4. The number of expectant parents attending group classes will increase by 50 percent in two years.

These are only a few of the nursing goals in the maternal and child health program. They do, however, illustrate the point being made. Each goal is stated in relation to the behavior that can be observed and measured, and gives definite direction to developing the plan of action.

The fact that any plan for a community must be viewed as valuable by the consumer has been noted many times throughout this book. Therefore, the goals toward which action is directed must also first and foremost be acceptable to the community, as well as being clearly defined and measurable.

One step toward a goal often depends upon another step. Thus, long-term goals are often based on a series of short-term goals. Establishment of a series of short-term goals gives community health nurses the opportunity to try or experiment with different mechanisms for change; to evaluate and measure their effectiveness toward reaching a long-term goal; and to make any changes necessary in future plans of action. For example, if the long-term goal for the future pattern of organization of nursing within a community is combination of services, one short-term goal might be to experiment first with combining services in just one area of the community. An evaluation of this goal will determine how combination of the remainder of the services might best be accomplished. It is easier to measure progress toward a short-term goal than toward a long-term goal. Evidence of progress gives a sense of accomplishment and satisfaction. The major value, however, is that the short-term goals are guideposts along the road toward meeting the long-term goals. As a result of evaluating the short-term goals, the appropriateness of the long-term goal can be evaluated.

In establishing both short- and long-term goals, the community health nurse must always keep in mind that nursing needs are only one part of a whole constellation of a community's other needs, and must be viewed in this context if they are to have any predictable chance for success.

Some of the short-term goals that are related to the long-term goal "All high-risk pregnant women will receive nursing supervision within 18 months" might be:

1. All high-risk pregnant women from the two largest hospital antenatal clinics will be referred for nursing supervision within six months.
2. Referrals for nursing supervision from nurses and physicians will increase by 10 percent within three months.
3. The number of expectant parents who utilize nursing supervision will increase by 25 percent in one year.

ALTERNATIVE ACTIONS FOR REACHING THE GOALS

Evaluation of alternative courses for reaching the desired goal or goals demands the very best skill and professional judgment of community health nursing. It involves making decisions and proposing and choosing alternative plans of action.

The following illustration will help to clarify the steps by which community health nursing decides on a plan of action in relation to one of the nursing goals it has established for a community. The goal was stated as "All high-risk pregnant women will receive nursing supervision within 18 months."

Classification of those who make up this high-risk group must be clearly understood and acceptable in order to avoid possible confusion and misunderstanding. What are some of the key factors which may account for this nursing need and may be preventing high-risk pregnant women from receiving nursing supervision? Are there enough facilities? Are they conveniently located? Are they utilized? Do the pregnant women know about the services which are available? Who refers them for nursing supervision? Do they view these services as valuable? Are there enough nursing personnel in the community to provide supervision? Are the nursing personnel adequately prepared? Are there enough financial resources? Are there problems unique to certain categories of these pregnant women?

Some key factors, identified on the basis of the foregoing questions, which account for this nursing need might be: lack of knowledge on the part of these women about either the value or availability of nursing supervision; few referrals from hospitals or other health resources; and minimal amount of nursing supervision provided in the areas with the greatest need.

Each of these factors which may prevent many high-risk pregnant women from receiving nursing supervision needs to be carefully studied in relation to the community. What might account for the fact that these women do not know about the value or availability of nursing supervision? What are the patterns of communication within this community? How might people get this kind of information? What is the educational level? What are the cultural patterns and attitudes toward health? What are the sources of health information? Is there an interagency referral system? What value do other health workers who might refer these women or inform them about nursing supervision place on this kind of care? What are the resources or mechanisms by which high-risk women might be better informed about the value and availability of nursing supervision?

After these factors have been identified and studied, consideration must be given to alternative plans of action. Some possible considerations might be to:

1. Develop a health education program for expectant mothers within the community which includes special attention to high-risk groups.
2. Plan a staff development program or workshop for community health nurses and other key health workers involved with high-risk pregnant women.
3. Organize neighborhood aides as outreach workers for high-risk pregnant women.
4. Develop an interagency referral system involving health professionals, groups, and institutions concerned with high-risk pregnant women.
5. Strengthen the sex-education and health-counseling programs within the junior high and the high school.

Priorities need to be developed for these possible alternative choices of action in order to determine which plan or combination of plans has the greatest chance of being the most effective and efficient in light of the particular community and its totality of resources.

In selecting the actions to reach the goals, consideration must be given to cost-effectiveness and to cost-benefit. Cost-effectiveness generally refers to a comparison of different ways of reaching the same objectives. It is a search for the most effectiveness at the lowest cost, and asks the question, How can we buy what we want at a lower cost? Costs are calculated, and alternative ways compared for achieving a specific set of results. The effectiveness may or may not be expressed in terms of dollars. Cost-benefit involves a comparison among several programs with differing objectives. It evaluates the monetary costs of a program in relation to the expected benefits to determine which is the best investment. It is often calculated as the benefit divided by the cost. The benefits are usually expressed in dollars. It is the most efficient way of using resources by relating the costs of a program to the expected benefits.

In referring to the alternative plans of action that were stated in relation to the long-term goal "All high-risk pregnant women will receive nursing supervision within 18 months," five alternative actions were proposed. Cost-benefit analysis would entail listing all of the possible benefits from each of the actions. Then the cost of each action would be calculated in terms of the monetary benefits. Selection of the action or actions would depend upon which gave the most benefit for the amount of money available. Cost-effectiveness analysis, in contrast to cost-benefit analysis, would not necessarily require a choice to be made between the actions as stated, but would be looking for the most effective way to reach the goal at the lowest price. Naturally, in this analysis, one also is interested in the benefits. However, in cost-efficiency analysis these are not necessarily expressed in relation to dollar amounts.

SELECTING THE ACTION FOR REACHING THE GOALS

After the alternative actions for reaching the goals have been identified, then the specific nursing actions should be selected. The difficulty in separating the steps of the planning process is evident, and a great deal of overlapping exists between establishing goals and deciding on ways in which they might best be reached. Although short- and long-term goals suggest directions for action, they do not designate the specific course of action. There are almost always several ways to get from one point to another. Considering alternatives and selecting the best way to reach the desired goal demands judgment based on knowledge, as well as creativity and imagination. For example, if development of an interagency referral system within a community is the goal of community health nursing, what is the best way to make this a reality? Would it be better to plan a workshop on referral for key people from all the agencies within the community who might be involved? Or would it be better to have a series of meetings with key people from each agency within the community? Or would it be better to meet with doctors, social workers, nurses, and others in individual groups? Or would it be better to try and develop a referral system between two agencies, evaluate the results, and then decide on next steps?

Different courses of goal-directed action must be considered and evaluated, and choices made in the light of each community's uniqueness and totality. The community itself, in the final analysis, holds the key to the success or failure of any plan of action.

In this chapter the process of planning to meet the nursing needs of the community has been explored and discussed. A plan, to be successful, must be realistic and clearly thought out as to goals, methods of accomplishment, and measurement. Equally important, it must be acceptable to the consumer and consistent with his whole way of life and his constellation of needs if it is to fulfill its purpose. Harnish aptly sums up the importance of planning when he says:

> We have come to a point in America where the atmosphere for planning has been built. But until such a time as our personal involvement in this process proves that giving up one's autonomy and that of one's organization in cooperative action is rewarding and self-fulfilling, we shall not make full use of the great potential found in the health professions of America for creating truly healthy communities.[5]

How well community health nursing can capture this essence of planning is a sign of its true professionalism.

Implementation and evaluation of the nursing plan of action are equally as important as its development. These are discussed in Chapter 14.

REFERENCES

1. U.S. Congress, *National Health Planning and Resources Development Act of 1974* (Public Law 93-164) Washington, D.C.: U.S. Government Printing Office, 1975).
2. N. Milio, "Health Care Organization and Innovation," *J. Health and Soc. Iss.* 12 (June 1971): 163.
3. National Commission on Community Health Services, *Health Is A Community Affair*, (Cambridge, Massachusetts: Harvard University Press, 1967), p. 2.
4. Ibid., p. 4.
5. T. I. Harnish, "Regional Medical Program Planning," *Amer. J. Public Health* 59 (March 1968): 770–20.

BIBLIOGRAPHY

Abel-Smith, B. "Cost Effectiveness and Cost benefit in cholera control." *WHO Chronicle* 27 (October 1973):407–9.

American Nurses' Association. *Standards of Community Health Nursing Practice.* Kansas City, Mo.: American Nurses' Association, 1973.

Conant, R. W. *The Politics of Community Health.* Report of the Community Action Studies Project. Washington, D.C.: Public Affairs Press, 1968.

Freeman, R. B. *Community Health Nursing Practice.* Philadelphia: W. B. Saunders Company, 1970.

Fifer, E. Z. "Hangups in Health Planning. *Amer. J. Public Health* 59 (May 1969): 765–69.

Fonaroff, A. "Identifying and Developing Health Services in a New Town." *Amer. J. Public Health* 60 (May 1970):821–28.

Griffith, E. I. "Where Do the VNA's Go from Here?" *Nursing Outlook* 16 (March 1968):29–31.

Harnish, T. T. "Regional Medical Program Planning." *Amer. J. Public Health* 59 (May 1969):770–72.

Henkel, B. O. *Community Health.* Boston: Allyn and Bacon, 1970.

Hilleboe, H. E. Editorial. "Concepts of Comprehensive Health Planning." *Amer. J. Public Health* 58 (June 1968):1011–13.

LeMontagne, M., and McKeehan, K. "Profile of a Continuing Care Program Emphasizing Discharge Planning." *J. Nurs. Admin.* 5 (October 1975):22–23.

Mattison, B. F. "Community Health Planning and the Health Profession." *Amer. J. Public Health* 58 (June 1968):1015–21.

Mott, B. F. J. "The Myth of Planning without Politics." *Amer. J. Public Health* 59 (May 1969):797–803.

Milio, N. "Health Care Organization and Innovation," *J. Health and Soc. Iss.* 12 (June 1971).

National Commission on Community Health Services. *Health Is a Community Affair.* Cambridge, Mass.: Harvard University Press, 1967.

National League for Nursing. *Planning, Providing, Fanancing Home and Community Health Services.* New York: National League for Nursing, 1972.

Novello, D. J. "The National Health Planning and Resources Development Act." *Nursing Outlook* 24 (June 1976):354–58.

O'Neil, C. E. "City-wide Planning for Nursing Service." *Nursing Outlook* 22 (September 1974):567–69.

Sanders, J. *The Community.* 3d ed. New York: Roland Press, 1974.

Scrutchfield, F. D. "Alternate Methods for Health Priority Assessment." *J. Comm. Health* 1 (Fall 1975):29–38.

Seder, R. "Planning and Politics in the Allocation of Health Resources. *Amer. J. Public Health* 63 (September 1973):747–77.

Silver, G. A. "What Has Been Learned About the Delivery of Health Services in the Ghetto?" In Norman, J. C., ed. *Medicine in the Ghetto.* New York: Appleton-Century-Crofts, 1969, pp. 65–72.

Simmons, H. J. III. "Community Health Planning—With or Without Nursing." *Nursing Outlook* 22 (April 1974):260–64.

Smith, W. T. "Cost Effectiveness and Cost Benefit Analysis for Public Health Programs." In Levey, S., and Loombs, N. P., eds. *Health Care Administration: A Managerial Perspective.* Philadelphia: J. B. Lippincott Company, 1975.

U.S. Congress. *National Health Planning and Resources Development Act of 1974.* (Public Law 94-164). Washington, D.C.: U.S. Department Printing Office, 1975.

U.S. Department of Health, Education and Welfare. *Planning for Nursing Needs and Resources.* Washington, D.C.: U.S. Government Printing Office, 1972.

Ziegler, D. "Overview of the Discharge Referral Planning Problem: What is Being Done Locally and Nationally?" In *Patient Discharge and Referral Planning—Whose Responsibility?* New York: National League for Nursing, 1974.

CHAPTER 14

IMPLEMENTING AND EVALUATING A NURSING PLAN OF ACTION FOR THE COMMUNITY

The implementation step of the nursing process is based upon the nursing plan for action as described in the previous chapter. The plan has clearly stated goals with measurable and/or observable outcomes. The goals have been mutually arrived at with consumers and the community health nurse; they are acceptable in relation to the norms and sanctions of the community; they are realistic and feasible; and they are congruent with the health priorities of the community and with other health plans in operation or pending. The plan is flexible and can be changed or altered as new information becomes available.

The people in any community have the ability to solve their own health problems. To do this, however, they must be involved in the very early stages of any plan which is developed. It is the people in the community who must make the final decisions about the priority of nursing needs, and the acceptable actions to meet the needs. In order to make these decisions, the consumers must have adequate information. This is where the community health nurse comes in. Through analysis of the data base, she provides the people with information about the health problems of their community. The people, in turn, provide the nurse with the information they have about the community, its people, and their desires, interests, and needs. In this sense, each is an expert in his own sphere.

The nurse and the persons most concerned determine together the nursing needs and future nursing actions. It is the people who have the final decision-providing power for the plan, the actions, and the implementation. The nurse has the responsibility to indicate the alternatives, and the consequences of each alternative. She then supports the decisions that are made, and works with the people to carry them out.

Community health nursing has a long history of working with the people in a community in developing nursing programs—in fact, this is one of the basic assumptions of community health nursing. Today, consumers are conserned about the kinds of health care available, and the cost of health services. With the mandate by the federal government for consumer participation in all aspects of health care, community health nurses are the best prepared professionals to take leadership in helping to solve community health problems. The community health nurse is one of the few health professionals who still visit people in their own homes, and who know first hand about their aspirations and needs. The people are apt to see the community health nurse as a friend and as a helping person, and thus will respond to her leadership in a positive way.

Implementation of the community nursing plan of action requires imagination, knowledge, judgment, and resourcefulness. It provides the nurse unlimited opportunities for innovation and creativity within a framework of reality. The sky may not always be the limit, but there are almost always ways to raise the ceiling. Flexibility is another necessary ingredient. A course of action may need redirecting or revising as a result of additional clues, inappropriate timing, new knowledge, new research, or evaluation. Implementation, therefore, demands commitment to priorities and goals, as well as flexibility.

Some of the questions the community health nurse might ask at this point are: Who are the people who will benefit most from the plan? What can they do to implement the plan? How can they see that it is nourished to fruition?

In implementing the plan, the community health nurse assumes many roles. Her foremost one will be a health advocate. She will also be a mobilizer of the people and of the resources; a cajoler when enthusiasm wanes; a provider of services; a role model; a teacher; an organizer and coordinator; a legislative instigator; and a communicator, to name a few. Her first contacts in mobilizing the people should be the persons who will benefit the most. They will form the nucleus for the further involvement of others in the community. A broad base of support is essential if the plan is to be sustained after the initial enthusiasm.

The information in the data base which is most important in implementing the plan relates to health facilities and resources, transportation, and channels of communication. The process of implementation includes the following steps:

1. ascertaining the resources
2. mobilizing the resources
3. activating the plan

ASCERTAINING THE RESOURCES

The first step in implementation is to ascertain the resources that are appropriate for the anticipated nursing actions. These may be the health-related facilities, such as hospitals, nursing homes, school health services, occupational health services, community nursing services, and so forth. The number of health professionals who work or live in the community should also be known. A basic question is: What organized community health nursing services are available?

Just as the health care system is complex, dynamic, and changing, so is the nursing care system within it. The fragmentation, instability, and individuality of contemporary nursing services make it unrealistic and even impossible at this time to suggest one best or most desirable nursing pattern. In reality, there are almost as many patterns as there are communities, and none is ideal. When implementing a nursing plan, we must look carefully at the network of services which make up the nursing care delivery system within the community. Nursing services are provided by various groups under different auspices. Some of the nurses providing the services are well prepared professionally, and others are less well prepared. Part of the nursing services are provided under the auspices of organized nursing, and part are under other auspices.

Nursing services may be provided by one agency, or a combination ot agencies. The patterns of community health nursing service most familiar are those provided by voluntary and official agencies. The Visiting Nurse Association, a voluntary organization, is primarily a nursing agency. The major thrust of its program is to provide nursing care on a part-time basis to individuals who are sick in their own homes. In providing services to the individuals who are sick, the health problems and nursing needs of the entire family are taken into consideration, with prevention of disease, promotion of health, and health teaching an inherent part of the program. However, the first priority for service is usually the bedside nursing needs of individuals.

The health department, an official agency, is organized according to the governmental structure of the locale. Thus, we find county health departments, city health departments, metropolitan health departments, regional health departments, and health departments for a single town or township. The community health nursing program is just one of several programs of the health department. More than half of the budgeted positions are for nurses. The major responsibilities of the nursing program within the health department are prevention and control of disease, health promotion, and health teaching for all groups. The activities of the nurse to carry out these responsibilities vary according to local conditions and facilities. Many of her activities consist of participation in clinics of various kinds, such as tuberculosis, venereal disease, well-child conferences, immunizations, multiphasic screening, family planning, mental retardation, antepartum, and postpartum. In some communities, school nursing is also her responsibility. Home visits are an integral part of these activities. Bedside nursing is not considered one of the major functions, but increasingly, the nursing programs in health departments are becoming certified as home health agencies.

In some communities, the nursing services of the health department and of the Visiting Nurse Association are provided separately, with little or no coordination. In other communities, organized structures have been established for the agencies to combine their services and to function as a combination agency.

The Council of Home Health Agencies and Community Health Services of the National League for Nursing has developed a proposed model for home health care benefits. A home health agency is defined as follows:[1]

> The term "home health agency" means a public or private agency or a subdivision of such an agency (including a home care department of a hospital), the need for which has been determined under "certificate of need" requirements.

It is further stated that a home health agency is

> primarily engaged in providing nursing, but also provides homemaker-home health aide services and at least one of the following services: physical therapy, occupational therapy, speech pathology service, nutrition, social work. Services should be available seven days a week.

Home health services have been defined as

> that component of comprehensive health care wherein services are provided to individuals and families in their places of residence for the purpose of promoting, maintaining, or restoring health or minimizing the effects of illness and/or disability. Services appropriate to the needs of the individual patient or family are planned, coordinated, and made available by an agency/institution (or a unit thereof) that is organized for the delivery of health care through the use of employed staff, contractual arrangements, or a combination of administrative patterns.

A growing proportion of nursing services are being provided by an increasing array of new and different kinds of agencies and organizations. For example, many hospitals have extended their services into the community through home care programs and satellite clinics. Some of the other services being offered are to special groups, such as mothers and children; and some are for particular areas of the community, such as specific neighborhoods. Categorized federal legislation for specific diseases, or for certain age groups, has resulted in a proliferation of special programs for selected persons who fit these categories. Attempts are being made to meet the multiple needs of people through multiservice agencies, neighborhood centers, and/or prepaid group insurance plans, to name a few. Many of the programs designed to meet multiple needs also include a nursing component. There are other new and exciting attempts to provide health care to the community through storefront clinics, mobile clinics, traveling vans, and family-life centers.

Community health nurses are involved in this kaleidoscope of programs in a variety of ways. The task of unraveling the fabric of the nursing care system from this crazy quilt for closer scrutiny is difficult. The nursing care system does not exist apart from the people who give it life and meaning—nurses and the growing army of nursing and health-related workers. Community health nursing must ascertain which personnel will be most effective in contributing to and carrying out the nursing plan of action. Most of this information has already been collected but needs to be scrutinized further. Some questions which should be asked are: How many community health nurses, both active and retired, are available to the community? What is their educational preparation and experience? How many are clinical specialists? Who has nurse practitioner skills? How many licensed practical nurses, home health aides, and nursing aides are there? How are these nursing and nursing-related personnel currently being utilized within the community? Are there nursing or multidiscipline teams in operation? What about nursing coordinators?

Knowledge about other health resources should include information that answers questions such as, Who uses what facilities and for what purposes—what are the patterns of utilization or nonutilization? Are there duplications and gaps in the available facilities and services? The available resources should also include the personnel who live and work in the community. Each community has a limitless reservoir of human potential from which to draw. Retired persons are taking an increasingly active role in community activities, and many have skills, knowledge, and interests in health and health-related areas. There are also persons in each community to whom the people turn for help prior to contacting a health professional. These indigenous persons, regardless of what their title may be, have for the most part been ignored by health professionals. Today, however, there is much discussion and some slight movement toward including these "primary health persons" in the mainstream of health care providers. This is another area in which community health nursing, because of its relationships with the people in the community, can identify these persons. It has an unheralded opportunity to demonstrate the contribution that can be made to health care by taking the leadership in working collaboratively with these persons who often perform "triage" functions in a community.

There are also organized groups in each community that should not be overlooked in ascertaining the resources and facilities. Often these groups receive little attention from the health professionals. However, as improvement of the health status of the community is a major goal of community health nursing, all of the groups should be considered as potential contributors toward this end. As mentioned previously, the wider the base of community support, the more effective any plan will be.

Transportation facilities and the mobility patterns of the people should be taken into consideration in the implementation of the nursing plan. Sometimes just changing the location of a clinic or a meeting place will increase participation because of the ease of getting there. Sometimes superhighways have bisected a community, which has changed the entire spectrum of who uses what services. This bisection has also changed the ways in which persons communicate with each other.

The formal and informal channels of communication have been discussed previously. Who communicates with whom and about what must be kept in mind in planning for implementation. Getting the approval of the community leaders is essential. How to get this approval will vary. It may be that these key persons will need to have some of their perceptions about health clarified and their ideas about health workers changed. This is where the early involvement of the people in the entire process will pay off, as they can interpret the nursing plan to community leaders.

Communication is the bridge by which people understand each other, teach, learn, and share ideas. Those who are involved in any action or venture want to know what is going on and want to be kept informed. Channels of communication among all who are to be involved in the nursing actions must be kept open. Collaboration means working together toward a common goal—nursing action. Coordination is the harmonious interaction of those equal in rank or importance. Coordination, therefore, unifies. Both collaboration and coordination necessitate mutual respect and understanding, and a willingness to seek and to give help. They mean free channels of communication, continuous dialogue, and a commitment to work together for what is best for the community.

Information about the current financial resources available to the community for the implementation of the plan is of utmost importance. Too often, however, money takes precedence over everything else, and many plans are never developed because there is no financial support in the offing. This approach is self defeating. When a nursing plan of action with clearly stated goals has been developed, then it is possible to seek funds for its implementation. There is no way funds can be solicited unless a plan has been developed. Vickers[2] would describe the developing of a plan and then the seeking of financial support as "goal-seeking" behavior. It is only with the successful seeking and completing of a goal that it can be decided if the goal was worth seeking. In contrast, if the plan is not developed because of the fear of no financial support, this would be described as threat-avoiding behavior. The goal was never attempted and thus it was never known if it was worth avoiding.

What sources can be tapped for funds? Are grant monies available from either the government or private sources? If only a portion of the necessary finances are available, what parts of the plan can be put off until a later date? What are the possibilities for fund raising in the community? These are a few of the questions that can be asked about funding for the nursing plan.

MOBILIZING THE RESOURCES

There is no one best way to mobilize the resources, as each community and its resources and facilities are different. We shall discuss some of the overall methods which have been found successful. In Chapter 11, the importance of having a representative group of consumers involved in the early stages was explored, and some suggestions were made about the composition of the group.

We have discussed each step of the nursing process as a separate entity in order to identify more clearly the many elements which must be considered. In reality, however, the steps are not discrete, and often each is going on simultaneously with much overlapping. Therefore, the original group has been involved in all phases, and the members are the key persons in the mobilization effort. They can serve as committee chairpersons, provide access to key persons in the community, clearly identify the groups whose sanction must be sought, and interpret other information about the community that can be known only by those who live there and know the way of life.

The community health nurse in a leadership position in the community is the focal person around which the plan will revolve. She can establish a mechanism for nurses in other leadership positions to meet together. As a group, they can determine how to combine their efforts to meet the nursing needs of the community, and to implement the nursing plan of action.

As the health advocate for the people, the community health nurse should be vocal and eloquent about the health problems and the factors that contribute to these problems. She should speak out about the high-risk groups in relation to health, and how the risks can be decreased. She should get involved wth community action groups that are interested in health. Through these activities, her role as a health advocate will become known.

Persons in strategic positions in the community should be contacted on a one-to-one basis about the nursing plan and what it means for the community. Such persons as the mayor, city or town manager, city council members, selectmen, board of supervisors, state legislators, and leaders of health and health-related agencies should be included in this category.

The persons who will be most affected by the plan should be organized and involved in all aspects of the mobilizing effort. Because of the benefits that will accrue to them, this group may be the most influential in making sure the plan is carried through.

A group that should not be overlooked by the community health nurse is the families that have been consumers of community health nursing services. They are often the best ones to interpret the nursing services to others.

Publicity about the nursing plan and the benefits to the community should be a continuous process. A television interview and spot radio announcements will help to keep the people informed. The newspapers also exert a great deal of influence. Invite a reporter to spend a day with you or one of your staff. He then can write a "day in the life of a community health nurse." Set up an information booth in a central spot in the community and have volunteers available to discuss the nursing plan and other health concerns.

Meet and discuss the nursing plan with organized health groups. The local medical society should be one of the priority groups with whom the nursing plan is discussed. In each community there are non–health-related organized groups which can make a contribution to the implementation of the plan. Church, fraternal, and social groups are examples.

In most communities there are also individuals and/or groups that have an uncanny ability to raise money, or to solicit supplies or donations where seemingly there was nothing. As the people become more and more involved, keep alert for those individuals and/or groups who can take responsibility to ferret out supplies and funds.

ACTIVATING THE NURSING PLAN

Mott has defined planning as follows: "Planning is an effort on the part of some group or organization to alter the behavior and conditions of other people. No matter how objective or wise the planners may be, they are engaged in deciding what is 'good' for other people and taking steps to obtain that good."[3]

Implementing the nursing plan of action in the community means changing the behavior and/or conditions of others. The nursing plan and goals are goal oriented, and stated in relation to the outcomes which can be measured or observed. Thus, change is inherent in the implementation of the plan. Change can be threatening and anxiety producing, as well as exciting and rewarding. It may mean a change in the role and responsibilities of nursing and other personnel; and a change in the allocation of funds for health. It will also mean a change in the health practices of the persons for whom the plan has been developed.

Warren,[4] in discussing change strategies in the community, has identified three situations. These include issue consensus, issue difference, and issue dissensus. Each situation requires a different strategy to bring about change.

Issue consensus situations are those in which there is general agreement by everyone concerned that the change is desirable. In other words, there is no question about the issue or issues. The only question revolves around how the change should be approached, who should be involved, some of the areas that should be included, and so forth. These are substantive aspects which lend themselves to solution by a strategy of *collaboration*. A discussion of these aspects and a pooling of the resources is the essence of this approach.

Issue difference relates to situations in which there may not be much opposition to the change, but neither is there much support. The approach here is to gain support for the change. There is an underlying assumption that if the real facts are known and understood, then the change will occur. This strategy comes under the heading of *campaign*. This is the stretegy that has been and still is used by public health workers. The bypassing of local and state health departments in some of the recent federal legislation may be due to the lack of success in the use of this strategy to change people's health behavior.

Issue dissensus refers to situations in which there is definite opposition to the change. Education about the issues and substance does not seem to have any effect. The strategy in this situation is one of *contest*. This strategy usually involves confrontation, heated debates, sit-ins, and other tactics which publicize the pros and cons and keep the issue before the public.

Keeping these strategies in mind is relevant in activating the nursing plan in the community. Which strategy will be most effective in a particular community? Is collaboration all that is required? Should it be supplemented with an educational campaign? Or is a more aggressive approach necessary to bring about a lasting change? Each situation must be looked at within the context in which the change is to take place. The power structure in the community must be analyzed, because in the final analysis the individuals, groups, or agencies that have the power will make the determination about the success or failure of the plan.

In the previous chapter, some alternative nursing actions were suggested for the goal "All high-risk pregnant women will receive nursing supervision within 18 months." One of the nursing actions was to strengthen the sex education and health counseling programs within the junior and senior high schools. The strategy for implementing this action will depend entirely upon the community in which it is to be implemented. Some of the questions that might be asked are: What do the school personnel know about a program of sex education? How do the parents feel about it? Do they see any difference between sex education and health counseling? Do the students want it? Will they utilize it? Who will determine the content? How will the community accept it? These are only a few of the questions that can be asked. The answers will help determine which approach will be most effective. As this subject is a controversial one in most communities, the approach may have to be different for each aspect of the implementation. The community health nurse must be cognizant of the prevailing mores and values in the community, and of where the power lies. Timing—when to use which approach—is vital, requiring the nurse to be constantly aware of the ebb and flow of the dynamics of the community.

There are also other ways to bring about nursing action. For example, a central registry of community health nurses might be organized in which the supply of nurses with education and experience in the various areas of community health nursing would be readily available. This would contribute to a more even distribution of educationally qualified community health nurses. It might also eliminate the present "piracy" of personnel by one agency from another, and make it less necessary to "rob Peter to pay Paul." Another community might employ a community health nurse practitioner who would have responsibility to ensure that the nursing needs of the community rather than the needs of the agencies would be the focus for nursing action in the community. Still another community might establish a coordinating council composed of representatives from organized nursing in the community, including hospitals, nursing homes, schools, industry, health department, Visiting Nurse Association, and other organizations employing nurses. In yet another community a coordinating council composed of nurses and consumers might be established.

EVALUATING THE NURSING PLAN FOR THE COMMUNITY

The final step in the process of community health nursing is the evaluation of the effectiveness of the plan of action which has been implemented in the community. There can be no justification for the existence of any plan or program without assurance of its effectiveness and value. Community health nursing programs which do not contribute to the solution of health problems in the community must be discarded or revised, or new ones developed.

The three approaches to evaluation—i.e., structure, process, and outcome—were discussed in Chapter 9. These approaches can also be used in evaluating a community health nursing program of any kind. The evaluation by structure applies to such elements as personnel, facilities, finances, and so forth. Process evaluation of the nursing plan in the community consists of the same elements that were discussed in the discussion of process evaluation in the family. The underlying assumptions are the same, whether the evaluation is applied to the family or to the community.

Outcome evaluation, steadily gaining stature, is the method of choice in evaluating the community health nursing plan or program. In outcome evaluation the focus is goal directed and evaluates the progress toward goal achievement. The goals must be stated in relation to outcomes which can be measured or observed—for example, the nursing goal which stated, "All high-risk pregnant women will receive nursing supervision within 18 months." One way to measure this goal would be to look at the number of high-risk pregnant women who are receiving nursing supervision at the end of 18 months and compare this number with those who were receiving this service at the beginning of the program. These numbers can be compared to the number of high-risk pregnant women in the community at each period of time.

The same kinds of questions that were asked about evaluation of outcomes in the nursing plan for the family should be asked about the nursing plan for the community. These questions were explored in Chapter 9.

Evaluation of the quality of care and of the services rendered by all health providers is of the highest priority today. Some of the reasons for the emphasis have been discussed throughout this book. Some of the methods being used to evaluate quality of care are: quality assurance; utilization review; nursing audit; accreditation; PSRO; and peer review.

Quality assurance refers to the criteria developed to evaluate the nursing actions, and the patient outcomes that are a result of the nursing actions.[5] Community health nurses are at the very beginning stage in the development of these kinds of criteria for quality assurance. The criteria for the nursing actions that are important for achieving patient outcomes must be developed by the community health nurses themselves. They must then develop the patient outcome criteria that will result from the nursing actions. For example, what are the essential nursing actions for women age 20 to 25 who are pregnant for the first time? What are the outcomes for this group of women that can be expected as a result of the nursing actions? Another example would be, What are the essential nursing actions for persons 60 years of age who have had a cerebral vascular accident and receive community health nursing services? What should be the results directly attributable to the nursing actions? The early stages of development of this method hold much promise for the evaluation of community health nursing services, as well as for other health services.

Utilization review is concerned with the services provided and with their relationship to patient need and agency objectives. The purpose is to improve service and ensure appropriate use of services rendered to individuals, families, and communities. It is a record review conducted by a committee which includes health professionals, consumers, and others knowledgeable in home health and community health services.[6]

Nursing audit is a method through which the quality of nursing care is assessed through a retrospective examination of records of patient care. It includes appraisal of care in relation to the individuality of the patient, as well as to the other and perhaps more easily assessed clinical dimensions of care. It provides quantifiable data from which generalizations about quality care can be made and action for improvement in quality can be planned.[7]

Accreditation of home health agencies and community nursing services is a joint venture by the National League for Nursing and the American Public Health Association. It is a voluntary process which determines whether an agency and its program have met rigorous criteria formulated by a committee of NLN's Council of Home Health Agencies and Community Health Services. On April 1, 1976, there were 73 accredited home health agencies and community nursing services.[8]

Peer review refers to the improvement of nursing care by nurses evaluating each other. The model developed by Gold and co-workers includes three steps: (1) the establishment of criteria for evaluation of nursing care by consensus of the persons involved, (2) a self-evaluation by each nurse using the criteria which have been developed, (3) a group review using the criteria which have been developed.[9]

Professional Service Review Organizations (PSRO) are required by federal legislation. They are a mechanism to evaluate the quality of medical care of hospitalized patients who are receiving services reimbursable by Medicare and Medicaid. Regional organizations have been established in many areas of the country. Services provided by physicians are the focus of the review. It is anticipated that services provided by nurses and other health providers will be included in the not-too-distant future.

Evaluation of the focus and emphasis of the nursing program within the community in relation to health maintenance, disease prevention, and health promotion, and of the priority accorded to each of these broad areas, helps to ensure a well-balanced program. If the major effort of a nursing program is directed toward bedside care, what happens to health promotion and disease prevention? Nursing priorities and programs must always be kept in balance.

Finally, the overall pattern by which community health nursing develops within a community needs to be studied in relationship to the trends and patterns of the broader community—regionalization, comprehensiveness, and finally, a national health plan. Thus, community health nursing must set its sights broadly and determine what and how it can best contribute to the promotion of the community's health. It must determine goals through which to make this contribution and continue to measure progress and accomplishment. This can be done only through evaluation.

Throughout Part II we have looked critically at each step of the process involved in community health nursing practice with the family as the patient, and again with the community as the patient. Irrespective of where the community health nurse works—in schools, in homes, with groups, in industry, in public health agencies, in ambulatory services, in neighborhood health centers, in a region, in a district, in a census tract, and so forth—the process is equally applicable. Although each situation in which she works will be different and the facts and content will vary, the process, which includes collecting and analyzing data, determining the health problems and identifying the nursing needs, determining the nursing care plan, and implementing and evaluating it, will remain essentially the same.

REFERENCES

1. Council of Home Health Agencies and Community Health Services. *Proposed Model for Home Health Care Benefits* (New York: National League for Nursing, 1976), p. 2.
2. G. Vickers, "What Sets the Goals in Public Health?" *New Engl. J. Med.* 258 (March 1958): 589–60.
3. B.J.F. Mott, "The Myth of Planning Without Politics," *Amer. J. Public Health* 59 (May 1969):797.

4. R.L. Warren, *The Community in America,* 2d ed. (New York: Rand McNally and Company, 1973), 382–88.
5. A. Watson and M. Mayers, "Evaluating the Quality of Patient Care Through Retrospective Chart Review," *J. Nurs. Admin.* 6 (March–April 1976):17–21.
6. National League for Nursing, *Utilization Review—Some Directions* (New York: National League for Nursing, 1973), p. 3.
7. M.C. Phaneuf, *The Nursing Audit: Profile for Excellence* (New York: Appleton-Century-Crofts, 1972), p. 1.
8. National League for Nursing. "Home Health Agencies and Community Services Accredited by NLN/APHA," *Nursing Outlook* 24 (April 1976):254–55.
9. E. Gold, *et al.* "Peer Review—A Working Experiment," *Nursing Outlook* 21 (October 1973):634–37.

BIBLIOGRAPHY

American Nurses' Association. *Standards of Community Health Nursing Practice.* Kansas City, Mo.: American Nurses' Association, 1973.

Bernal, H. "Power and Interorganizational Health Care Projects." *Nursing Outlook* 24 (July 1976):418–21.

Brichner, P. W., *et al.* "Outreach to Welfare Hotels, the Homebound, the Frail." *Amer. J. Nurs.* 76 (May 1976):762–64.

Council of Home Health Agencies and Community Health Services. *Proposed Model for Home Health Care Benefits.* New York: National League for Nursing, 1976.

Ellwood, P. M. *Assuring the Quality of Health Care.* Minneapolis: Inter Study, 1973.

Gold, E., *et al.* "Peer Review—a Working Experiment." *Nursing Outlook* 21 (October 1973):634–37.

Helt, E. H., and Pelikan, J. A. "Quality Medical Care's Answer to Madison Avenue." *Amer. J. Public Health* 65 (March 1975):284–90.

Howell, J. R., Osterweis, M., and Huntley, R. R. "Curing and Caring—a Proposed Method for Self-Assessment in Primary Care Organizations." *J. Comm. Health* 1 (Summer 1976):256–75.

Kane, R. L., *et al.* "Measuring Outcomes of Care in an Ambulatory Primary Care Population." *J. Comm. Health* 1 (Summer 1976):233–40.

Kissinger, C. L. "Quantifying Nursing Utilization." *J. Nurs. Admin.* 3 (January/February, 1973):35–40.

Mott, B. J. F. "The Myth of Planning without Politics." *Amer. J. Public Health* 59 (May 1969):797–803.

Murphy, M. J. "The Development of a Community Health Orientation Scale." *Amer. J. Public Health* 64 (December 1975):1293–96.

———*Accreditation of Home Health Agencies and Community Nursing Services. Policies and Procedures.* New York: National League for Nursing, 1976.

———"Home Health Agencies and Community Nursing Services Accredited by NLN?" *APHA, April 1976. Nursing Outlook* 24 (April 1976):254–55.

——— *Type, Length and Cost of Care for Home Health Agencies.* New York: National League for Nursing, 1975.

——— *Utilization Review–Some Directions.* New York: National League for Nursing. 1973.

National League for Nursing. *Utilization Review—Some Directions.* New York: National League for Nursing, 1973.

Phaneuf, M. *The Nursing Audit: Profile for Excellence.* New York: Appleton-Century-Crofts, 1972.

Price, J., and Vincent, P. "Program Evaluation: What to Ask before You Start." *Nursing Outlook* 24 (February 1976):84–87.

Roos, N. P. "Evaluating Health Programs: Where Do We Find the Data?" *J. Comm. Health* 1 (Fall 1975):39–51.

Vickers, G. "What Sets the Goals in Public Health?" *New Engl. J. Med.* 258 (March 1958): 589–96.

Warren, R. L. *The Community in America.* 2d ed. New York: Rand McNally & Company, 1973.

Watson, A., and Mayers, M. "Evaluating the Quality of Patient Care through Retrospective Chart Review.' *J. Nurs. Admin.* 6 (March–April 1976):17–21.

CHAPTER 15

THE ROAD AHEAD

The best of times can also be the worst of times. Supersonic planes booming over traffic-clogged highways; tree-lined suburbs and decaying inner cities; zooming salaries, soaring prices, and endless welfare lines; exploding knowledge and pervading illiteracy; more and more people for fewer and fewer jobs; democracy and civil-rights demonstrations. This is America in the last quarter of the twentieth century. Dynamism, change, and contrast have always been characteristic of this country. It has from the very beginning been tempered and molded by struggle, strife, and turmoil. Today, however, the tempo of change is accelerating at a geometric rate, with more people, more cars, more demonstrations, and multiplying problems.

The health care delivery system is equally chaotic and on the threshold of a massive reorganization. One cannot predict just what kind of system is evolving, but no one will deny that dramatic revisions are in process. The current health care system, which is rightfully referred to as a nonsystem, is characterized by specialization, fragmentation, and proliferation, with resulting gaps and duplication; crisis orientation, with lack of long range planning; complexity and automation, with resulting depersonalization. The time has come when the American people will no longer tolerate this kind of care with its escalating costs and inadequate services. Their rising expectations and increasingly insistent demands for more readily available and more effective health care have been to some avail, with discernible organizational patterns gradually coming into focus. No one is clear about exactly what form they will take, but the following are examples of some of the elements or characteristics predictable at this time:

1. Services will be provided by a multidiscipline team. Many health professionals and consumers will be involved as members of the health team.
2. Services will be comprehensive, with a variety of prepaid group insurance plans, comprehensive neighborhood health centers, and health maintenance organizations.
3. Care outside the hospital will receive greater emphasis, with provisions for services to people wherever they are.
4. Patient care facilities will be increasingly automated and complex due to the knowledge explosion and scientific and technologic developments.
5. The providers of care will be held responsible and accountable to the consumer for the quality of health services received.
6. Health care will be organized in such a way that entrance into it and orderly progression within it will be facilitated.
7. A national health insurance plan will become a reality, although its form and structure are unclear at present. Undoubtedly, health will finally become a public utility.

The period of transition between the present chaotic nonsystem and an emerging system of health care will be painful and exciting. Rapid changes are occurring, with old patterns, methods, and long traditions being shattered and new ones emerging, but not as yet stabilized. This is an era in which nothing will remain static for any length of time, and decisions made today may not be valid tomorrow. Community health nursing, with other professional groups, is part of this scene. Its future in this changing milieu is still uncertain. How it responds will either make it a potent force in shaping the health care system or consign it to oblivion. We believe that community health nursing is responding to societal needs, and we are optimistic about its future.

No professional group shapes its own destiny, but it can take advantage of the available opportunities to determine the directions in which it should go. The evolution of community health nursing is dotted with periods of crisis and uncertainty. It has responded at some times by assuming leadership and forging ahead; and at others by marking time and maintaining the status quo. It is risky to predict what its future holds. However, we believe it has the elements and the potential for making a significant contribution to society if it utilizes its wisdom, energy, and creativity to harness these assets for maximum effectiveness.

Community health nursing has a vast storehouse of knowledge about health problems of families and communities, and an awareness, gained from long experience, about their hopes and aspirations. From the beginning its locus of operation has been the community, and its main focus has been the relationship of the health of the family to the health of the community. Community health nursing is taking more initiative in sharing its knowledge and concerns with others, and in assuming leadership in mobilizing appropriate persons and resources for social action for health. It is becoming increasingly astute and knowledgeable about the politics of power, sources of money, and legislative channels of government. It is already having legislative input at the national and state level and is contributing its know-how to help bring about needed changes in community health. It encompasses the largest group of community health workers and has the ability and experience to provide real leadership toward improved health.

The consumer is very much involved in the determination of the kind and quality of services he wants and needs. Increasingly, federal legislation will continue to require significant consumer involvement in all federally funded health planning. Community health nursing will continue to work with citizens and other professionals in planning and implementing health programs, and in sharing its knowledge and experience with other professional groups. It will also be held accountable to the consumer for assuring that he receives quality care.

One of the results of the knowledge explosion is, and will continue to be, an even greater increase in specialization of health workers, with each concentrating on one aspect of health in the individual or the community. Specialism will also invade community health nursing, and its expertise will be built on the concepts of the family and the community as the patient. Thus, the community health nurse's practice will be geared to a broad generalist approach, and she might well be defined as a "generalized specialist." By building upon the skills she already has and developing further expertise, the community health nurse can help families integrate the services they are receiving. The impression that in these days one goes to one physician or health facility for a left foot, and to another for a right ear, is not too far from the truth. One might ask who really is concerned about the whole patient—much less the whole family. The fragmentation which has resulted from specialization is frightening and potentially hazardous. Never was the need for a generalist more pressing—and the community health nurse can fill that need.

The community health nurse practitioner will provide leadership in assessing and determining the health problems of the community and in mobilizing the health resources. These practitioners will collaborate with other nurses. They will provide leadership and consultation to the growing numbers of nurses giving increasingly complex nursing care to sick people at home, and will help them to identify health problems of the family in addition to the illness of its members. Disease prevention health, promotion, and maintenance of health as the focus of community health nursing will become more pronounced in the future.

As we look ahead at the shape of things to come and consider the possible directions and potential contribution of community health nursing within this evolving health system, we believe that it will become the professional group which will provide primary health care to families. It has always assumed part of this responsibility and has considerable knowledge and experience as a basis for further development of this role. Community health nursing is already carrying out many of the functions once thought to be those of the general practitioner. For example:

1. It has long assessed the health needs of individuals within the family, and of the family as a whole.
2. It has made judgments about whether medical care is needed, what kind, and where it is to be obtained.
3. It has coordinated various health services and interpreted medical orders.
4. It has helped to improve health practices of the family and has prescribed time-tested remedies.
5. It has recognized the value of cultural and ethnic practices and has exploited these to the advantage of the families.
6. It has intervened and supported families during periods of stress and crisis.

These and many other long-standing activities of community health nursing are being legitimized. Increasingly, community health nursing is adding additional knowledge and skills to its armamentarium, such as:

1. clarifying the independent functions of the nurse, as well as her dependent and interdependent functions
2. adding skills, previously considered the prerogative of the physician, such as taking the health history and physical assessment of individuals.
3. becoming skillful in making judgments about the medical care and treatment a family needs and in prescribing some of the diagnostic tests basic to determining the appropriate point of entry into the medical-care system
4. developing greater depth of knowledge about growth and development of individuals, and the common ailments of various age groups

With this and other appropriate knowledge, the community health nurse practitioner can now more effectively develop her own role. These added responsibilities are all logical extensions of nursing. Community health nurse practitioners are now better prepared than before to work in a peer relationship with the multidiscipline health team.

In order for the emerging health care system to be effective, the education of health workers will undergo a metamorphosis. No longer will each discipline educate its practitioners in isolation without regard to the changing roles and responsibilities of other professionals. A common core of knowledge necessary for every health worker will be identified, and core courses and curriculum plans will be developed. This will provide an opportunity for students in health-related programs to be educated together and to understand each other's contributions. By having a common core of knowledge, students will also be able to change their career choices without being penalized by having to start their education all over again.

With a core curriculum it will be even more important than it is now for each discipline to identify its contribution to health care and to demonstrate its value. This is as true of nursing and community health nursing as of all other disciplines. If nursing is to become a full-fledged partner of the health team, its members must have equal educational preparation. In this tecnologic era with its high premium on education, an apprentice-type preparation for professional practice will no longer suffice. Nursing must move into the mainstream of higher education in order to realize its full potential in the current decade.

The decade ahead will continue to be a period of experimentation with various educational programs. The demand for upward mobility, nontraditional programs, part-time and extramural learning, and awarding of college credit for nonacademic experiences will continue. We believe that provision of diverse and creative learning opportunities will increase—but that a strong nursing core, within a theoretic framework, will remain basic to the education of the professional nurse. The possibility that professional nursing education will become a post-baccalaureate pursuit, like training for medicine and social work, is on the horizon.

Undoubtedly, there will be different licensure examinations for graduates of varying types of educational programs, and mechanisms for interstate mobility will be worked out. The American Nurses' Association will have a greater role in credentialing practitioners for competence.

Programs to educate nurses for expanded and extended roles are well accepted and will become part of the system of graduate education for nurses, with generally accepted standards for admission and graduation.

Due to a variety of factors, such as age shifts in the population and the average age of teachers who are now employed, there will be fewer job opportunities for teachers now and in the next decade. Consequently, there will be an abundance of young people and college graduates, both male and female, who may be attracted into the health field. Many of these will wish to select nursing as a career. The impact of this phenomenon on the expansion of baccalaureate programs is unclear at this time. Undoubtedly, there will be more men in it, and larger numbers of these men will be in administrative positions—this has happened in other "women's professions" of which men have become a part.

Specialized programs on the graduate level will continue to increase. The continuous generation of new knowledge through science, technology, and research necessitates the constant reevaluation of content in graduate and baccalaureate programs for its relevance to nursing practice.

The need for continuing education for all professions is undeniable. Continuing education for all practicing nurses will be required, and monitoring mechanisms will be established.

There is urgent need for research in nursing—research in relation to clinical practice, education, nursing-care delivery systems, and basic nursing theory—so that we will be able to better determine what we do that makes a difference, and in order to discover other and better ways to care for patients. Whatever the reasons may be for the paucity of clinical research to date, the road ahead looks more promising. Renewed interest in and concern for clinical practice, with accompanying expansion of specialized graduate nursing programs, has resulted in a growing reservoir of well-prepared and highly motivated nurses. Doctoral programs in nursing will increase as more basic nursing theory is developed. The graduates of doctoral programs will join the nurse practitioners and clinical specialists in bringing a new focus and commitment, as well as knowledge and skill, to their particular fields of interest. The community health nurse specialist is part of this group.

Nursing has an increasing pool of practitioners with a higher level of education—more with doctorates, more with master's degrees in a variety of specialty areas, and increasing numbers prepared at the baccalaureate level. This growing reservoir of knowledgeable men and women is already having a favorable impact on nursing and continues to be a hope for the future in helping to solve some of the persistent problems in nursing, nursing organizations, nursing education, and, ultimately, the health of the people.

Because the community health nurse specialist—it is hoped, the community health nurse practitioner of the future—is closely involved in caring for the patient and his family, she will continue to be in a strategic position to identify nursing problems that need to be studied. In order to improve practice, she will identify and document what she is doing, develop and test hypotheses, and contribute to theories for nursing practice. Many of the nursing problems in the home seem to be different from those in the hospital, but are they? How is effectiveness of nursing intervention measured? What nursing decisions are made by the nurse, and what is the effect on the family? Are the community patterns for providing nursing care effective? How can this be measured? These are only a few examples of the kinds of questions which will need to be raised and for which answers must be sought. When there are specialists in community health nursing, it is much more likely that problems in practice will be identified, and research initiated.

No one will deny that community health nursing has a great deal of hard work ahead—to improve its practice, its system of delivering care, and its education. It has, however, already come a long way and through other anxious periods of history. Community health nursing will continue to evolve and change. It will continue to be influenced by an interplay of societal forces and to be a force in itself. It is because of this dynamism of the world in which we live that in this book we have focused on the process of community health nursing, as this process will remain essentially unchanged in a changing world. There are exciting times ahead. Community health nursing has the potential to make a contribution to the health of the people. We believe it also has the wisdom, energy, and creativity.

BIBLIOGRAPHY

DeLoughery, G. L., and Gebbie, K. M. *Political Dynamics.* St. Louis: The C. V. Mosby Company, 1975.

Kramer, M. *Reality Shock.* St. Louis: The C. V. Mosby Company, 1974.

Novello, D. J. "The National Health Planning and Resources Development Act." *Nursing Outlook* 24 (June 1976)354–58.

Toffler, A. *Future Shock.* New York: Bantam Books, 1974.

U.S. Congress. *National Health Planning and Resources Development Act of 1974* (Public Law 93-174). Washington, D.C.: U.S. Government Printing Office, 1975.

U.S. Department of Health, Education and Welfare. *Nurse Training—Title VIII—Public Health Service Act.* DHEW Publication No. (HRA) 76-42, 1975.

Wise, H., Beckhard, R., Rubin, I., and Kyte, A. *Making Health Teams Work.* Cambridge, Mass.: Ballinger Publishing Company, 1974.

APPENDIX A
FAMILY DATA COLLECTION

Name of family____________________________________

Address ____

I. Family Characteristics

A. Persons living in the household

Name	Date of Birth	Sex	Race	Relation to Head of House	Occupation

B. Members of family not living in household

C. Occupational history of each adult member

D. Roles of members—what are assigned household tasks?

Adults

Children

E. Relationships of members—how do they get along?

Husband-wife

Father-children

Mother-children

Children-children

F. Decision making—who makes decisions? How?

Major decisions

Minor decisions

G. Sleeping arrangements

Which family members sleep together?

Which family members sleep alone?

What type of bed does each have?

What are the usual hours of sleep? Bedtime Arising Rest periods

Adults

Children

H. Eating patterns

Observations about kitchen and mealtimes

Observations of family members for nutritional status

24-hour family-food intake beginning with previous day's breakfast

Breakfast

Lunch

Dinner

Snacks

I. Leisure—what are the usual activities?

Adults

Children

II. Socioeconomic and Cultural Factors

A. Educational level—what is the highest school grade completed?

Adults

Children

B. Ethnic group background

C. Religious affiliation

D. Occupation of working members

E. Income

Family income $______ (week, month, year)

Source—Salary $______ Savings $______ Investments $______
Pensions $______ Social Security $______ Veterans $______
AFDC $______ Welfare $______
Other $ ______________________________

Contributions of working members
Member ____________ Amount $ __________ (week, month, year)

Are expenses greater, less than, or equal to income?
greater less equal

Who plans how the money is spent?

F. Social relations—whom do the family members interact with outside the immediate family, and what community activities do they participate in?

Extended family ______________
Neighbors ______________
Friends ______________
Church ______________
Clubs ______________
Community activities (list) ______________
____
Other ______________

G. Value system

Observations of nurse

Home ______
Furniture ______
Neighborhood ______
Other ______

Comments by mother or other family members

III. Environmental Factors

A. Housing

Type ______ Own ______ Rent ______
Number of rooms ______ Furniture adequate ______ inadequate ______
Type of refrigeration for food ______
Toilet facilities—inside ______ outside ______
Water supply—municipal ______ well ______ other ______
Flies—yes ______ no ______
Accident hazards (list)

B. Neighborhood

Residential ______ industrial ______ rural ______
urban ______ ghetto ______ suburban ______ other

Type of dwellings

Condition of dwellings

Accessibility of play areas—Yes No

Accessibility of health facilities—Yes No
(list)

Accessibility of churches—Yes No

Accessibility of schools—Yes No

C. Transportation

Public transportation—Yes No
Adequate Yes No
Other

IV. Health and Medical History

A. Present illnesses of each member

B. Is any family member taking any medication—Yes No
If "yes," name of drug, how often taken, and by whom?

C. History of past significant illnesses and accidents of each member

D. Immunization status of each member

E. What is the state of dental health of each member?

F. Physical assessment of each member as indicated
Head
Neck
Face
Eyes
Ears
Nose and sinuses
Mouth and throate
Skin
Breasts
Heart
Lungs
Abdomen
Back
Extremities
Genitals

G. How is medical care financed?

Medical insurance __________ Medicare __________
Hospital insurance __________ Medicaid __________
Own finances __________ Other __________

H. What is the knowledge and attitude of the family about health?

I. What does the family perceive as its health problems?

J. What does the nurse perceive as the family health problems?

K. What has been the previous experience of the family with the community health nurse? What did she do?

L. What does the family think is the reason for present visit by the nurse?

M. What are the nursing needs as seen by the family?

N. What is the family's expectation of the community health nurse?

O. How has the family managed in previous situations of illness or crisis?

Own resources ____________________
Extended family ____________________
Other relatives ____________________
Friends ____________________
Neighbors ____________________
Significant others ____________________
Other ____________________

P. How will family manage between visits of community health nurse?

V. Summary

A. What are the family health problems (list with priorities)

B. To which of the family health problems can nursing make a contribution? (nursing needs)

C. Which of the family nursing needs will you give first priority? Second priority? Third priority? And so forth.

APPENDIX B

COMMUNITIY NURSING SURVEY GUIDE

Community________________________ Date of Survey ________________________

I. **The Community**

A. Description: Include general identifying data, i.e., location, topography, climate, urban, rural, etc.

B. Boundaries: Specific boundaries surrounding study area

C. Area in square miles

D. Type of government (mayor, city manager, board of supervisors, etc.)

E. History: Include significant changes such as urban development, major highway construction, regionalization, shifts in industry.

F. Community changes anticipated

II. **Population Characteristics**

A. Total population for 19______ (last census)

B. Population changes in last 10 years

C. Population per square mile

D. Mobility of population

E. Population and age distribution

	COMMUNITY				STATE		NATIONAL	
Age group	**Current Popula- tion 19____**	**per- cent**	**Popula- tion 10 years ago**	**Per- cent**	**Popula- tion**	**Per- cent**	**Popula- tion**	**Per- cent**
0–5								
5–14								
15–24								
25–34								
35–44								
45–54								
55–64								
65–74								
75+								

F. Sex and race distribution—19________

		COMMUNITY	STATE	NATIONAL
Race	**Sex**	**Number/Percent**	**Number/Percent**	**Number/Percent**
Nonwhite	Female			
	Male			
White	Female			
	Male			
Total				

G. Ethnic group composition—19________

	COMMUNITY	STATE	NATIONAL
Race	**Number/Percent**	**Number/Percent**	**Number/Percent**

H. Religious distribution—19________

	COMMUNITY	STATE	NATIONAL
Religion	**Number/Percent**	**Number/Percent**	**Number/**Percent
Catholic			
Protestant			
Jewish			
Other			

I. Educational levels (persons 25+) 19________

	PERCENT OF POPULATION		
Education	**Percent**	**Percent**	**Percent**
No Schooling			
1–4 Years			
5–8 Years			
Attended High School			
Graduate from High School			
Attended College			
Median Years of Education			

J. Socioeconomic characteristics

1. Income of families—19________

	PERCENT OF FAMILIES		
	COMMUNITY	STATE	FEDERAL
Income	**Percent**	**Percent**	**Percent**
Under $3,000			
$3,000–5,999			
$6,000–9,999			
$10,000+			
Median Income			

2. Leading industries

Name	Address	No. Employed

3. Occupations (list categories)

4. Estimated level of unemployment

Community ____________ State ____________ National ____

III. **Environmental Factors**

A. General description of environment

B. Housing

1. Condition of housing

TYPE OF DWELLING	GOOD No./Percent	FAIR No./Percent	POOR No./Percent

2. Ownership and rental status

Units owned (%) ____________________
Units rented (%) ____________________

C. Sanitation

1. Water supply, sewage, trash, and garbage

	Public	**Private**
Source of Water Supply	____________	____________
Sewage Disposal	____________	____________
Trash and Garbage	____________	____________

D. Protection

1. Fire protection (describe) ______________________________
2. Police protection (describe) ____________________________
3. Environmental surveillance or monitoring ________________
4. Safety (describe significant safety programs or hazards)
   ____
   ____

E. Transportation

Describe transportation systems: bus, suburban train, air, private automobile, other

F. Other significant environmental factors

IV. Communication Resources

A. News Media
Newspapers

Name	**Publication Schedule**	**Circulation**
____________	____________	____________
____________	____________	____________
____________	____________	____________

B. Radio stations (local)

C. Television

D. Key community leaders and/or decision makers (list and identify)

E. Other

V. Health Information

A. Vital statistics

19______

	COMMUNITY	STATE	NATIONAL
	Number/ Rate	Number/Rate	Number/Rate
Live births			
Neonatal deaths			
Infant deaths			
Maternal deaths			
Deaths			

D. Disease incidence and prevalence

19______

	COMMUNITY	STATE	NATIONAL
Disease	Number/Rate	Number/Rate	Number/Rate
	I P I P	*I P I P*	*I P I P*
Cardiovascular			
Cancer			
Diabetes			
Other significant			

C. Leading causes of death*

	COMMUNITY		STATE	NATIONAL
Cause of Death	Number	Rate	Rate	Rate
1.				
2.				
3.				
4.				
5.				
6.				
7.				
8.				
9.				
10.				

**Include other information and/or statistics significant for your community and compare with state and national figures.*

VI. Health Facilities and Resources

A. Hospitals
Name
1) Ownership
2) Accreditation, type
3) Average length of hospitalization

Type of Service

medical	________	psychiatric	________
surgical	________	communicable disease	________
maternity	________	intensive care	________
pediatric	________	chronic disease	________
rehabilitation	________		

B. Nursing homes

Name

Ownership ________
Accreditation ________
Certification ________
Bed capacity ________
Services ________
Other ________

C. Ambulatory Services

Name of hospital or clinic

Emergency	________	Drug Addiction	________
Maternity	________	Alcoholism	________
Pediatric	________	Psychiatric	________
Family Planning	________	Dental	________
Medical	________	Eye	________
Surgical	________	Other	________
Orthopedic	________		

D. Other health care resources

1. Occupational health services

2. School health services

3. Health departments

4. Voluntary health agencies

5. Comprehensive health centers (neighborhood centers, Maternal & Infant, Children & Youth, etc.)

6. Prepaid group health plans

7. Other

E. Health-related planning groups (e.g., Health Service Agencies (HSAs), Neighborhood Councils, etc.)

Briefly describe purpose, people served, personnel of these resources, and services provided to the community.

F. Health personnel

Personnel	No. Living in Community	No. Active
Physician		
Dentist		
Registered Nurse		
Licensed Practical Nurse		
Physical Therapist		
Sanitary Engineers		
Social Workers		
Occupational Therapists		
Significant Others		

VII. **Community Health Nursing Services***

A. Identifying data

1. Name of agency

2. Purpose of agency

**This section of guide may need to be modified to meet local community differences.*

3. Legal authority

4. Certified Home Health Agency Yes No
   Date of certification

5. Accredited (APHA-NLN) Yes No
   Date accredited

6. Organization: (describe and/or include Table of Organization)

7. Administration
   (1) Board of Directors
      a. Number of board members Total M F
      b. Community groups or interestsrepresented (list)
      c. Maximum number of consecutive terms possible for a board member
      d. Frequency of general board meetings
      e. Regular addendance at board meetings by Nursing Director Yes No
      f. Committees of the board (list)

   (2) Nursing Director
      a. Job description

      b. Lines of authority

B. Finances

1. Income
   Capital funds and endowment
   Tax funds (list sources)

   Earnings
   Fees from patients ______________
   Insurance ______________
   Medicare ______________
   Medicaid ______________
   Welfare ______________
   Other ______________

   All other income (grants, refunds, etc.)

   Total Income

2. Expenditures
   Salaries
   Director ______________
   Supervisor ______________
   Assistant Supervisor ______________

Consultants
  Nursing ____________
  Nonnursing ____________
Clinical Nurse Specialist ______
Community Health Nurse ______
Registered Nurse ____________
Liecensed Practical Nurse ______
Home Health Aide ____________
Neighborhood Aide ____________
Clerical ____________
Other ____________

Staff Development ____________
Transportation ____________
Nursing Supplies and Equipment ____________
Rent and Related Expenses ____________
Office Expenses (records, telephone, etc.) ____________
All other general expenses (specify) ____________

Total Expenses ____________

3. Method used to determine cost per unit

Date
Cost per visit
Charge for visit Date established

C. Personnel

1. Professional nursing personnel

	No.	Educ. Prep.	Total Experience CHN	Length of Experience with Agency	Part-Time	Full Time
Executive Director						
Supervisor						
Assistant Supervisor						
Nurse Consultants						
Clinical Specialist (specify area)						
Practitioners (specify area)						
Registered Nurses						
Others (list)						

2. Other professional personnel

	No.	Educ. Prep.	No. of Years with Agency	Full Time	Part Time
Physician					
Physical Therapist					
Occupational Therapist					
Social Worker					
Statistician					
Nutritionist					
Sanitarian					
Health Educator					
Others (list)					

3. Other personnel*

	No.	No. of Years with Agency	Full Time	Part Time
Licensed Practical Nurse				
Home Health Aide				
Neighborhood Aide				
Clerical Staff				
Other (list)				

4. Volunteers

No. of hours of assistance available last year —19______
Activities carried by volunteers (list)

5. Utilization of personnel

a. Describe responsibility of staff
b. Rationale for nursing responsibilities
c. Job descriptions

**Indicate type of responsibilities*

D. Services

1. Total cases   Visits   in 19______
2. Care of the sick

Classification of Illness	Cases	Visits	Percentage of Total Visits
Cancer			
Heart Disease			
Diabetes			
Others (list)			
Tuberculosis			
Venereal Disease			
Other Communicable Diseases (list)			

3. Health Guidance

Classification	Cases	Visits	Percentage of Total Visits
Maternity Antepartal			
Postpartal			
Infant Premature			
Neonatal other than Premature			
Other—1 Year			
Preschool			
School			
Adult			
Adult 65 +			

4. Clinic service

Type of Clinic	No. Sessions per Month	Attendance per Session	Total Monthly Attendance	Nurses per Session	Other Personnel per Session

5. School health service

Type of School	No. of Schools	Pupil Enrollment	No. of Teachers
Kindergarten			
Nursery			
Elementary			
Secondary			
Special Ed.			
Day Care Centers			
Head Start			
Total			

6. Comprehensive Health, Neighborhood Health, or Health Maintainance Organization (describe nursing program)

7. Other services
   Identify and describe other nursing services and/or programs involving Community Health Nursing, such as those relating to Occupational Health, Family Planning, Drug Addiction, Alcoholism, Community Mental Health, Parent Teaching, or other.

E. Referrals and contracts

1. Sources of referral for community health nursing

   Hospitals (including OPD)
   Home Care Programs
   Prepaid Group Plans
   Other Agencies
   Family or Patient
   Friend
   Community Health Nurse
   Other (indicate)

2. System for referral between community health nursing services within the community (describe)

3. Contractual agreements with other community agencies for community health nursing services (identify and describe)

VIII. **Summary**

A. What are the health problems indicated by the data base? (List in order of priority).

B. Identify the nursing need for each health problem (contribution of nursing to the solution).

C. Which of the nursing needs should be given first priority, second priority, third priority, etc? (List.)

INDEX